INTERNAL MEDICINE

Mastering the Boards and Clinical Examinations

RESPIROLOGY

A.B.R. Thomson

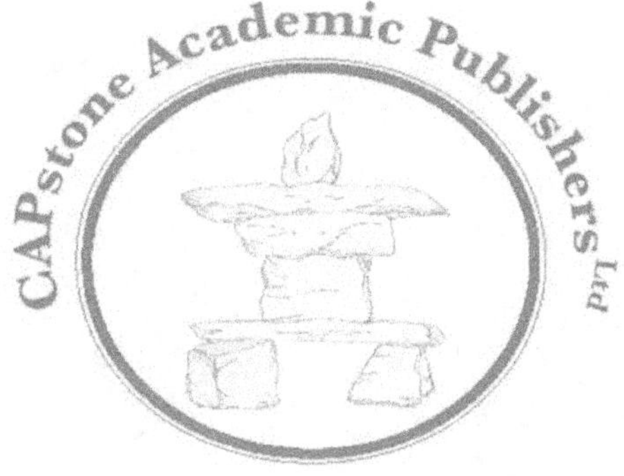

CAPstone (Canadian Academic Publishers Ltd) is a not-for-profit company dedicated to the use of the power of education for the betterment of all persons everywhere.

"The Democratization of Knowledge"

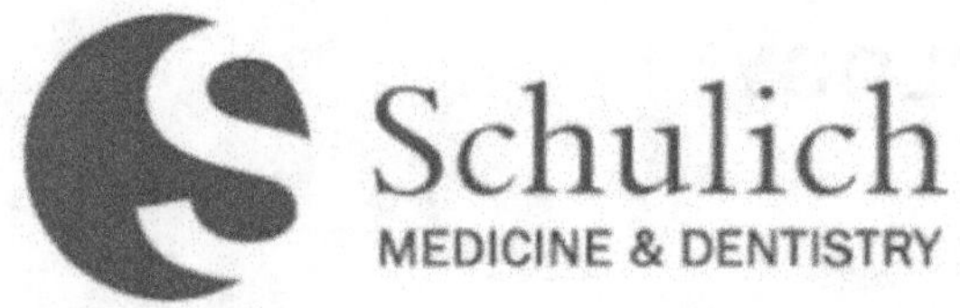

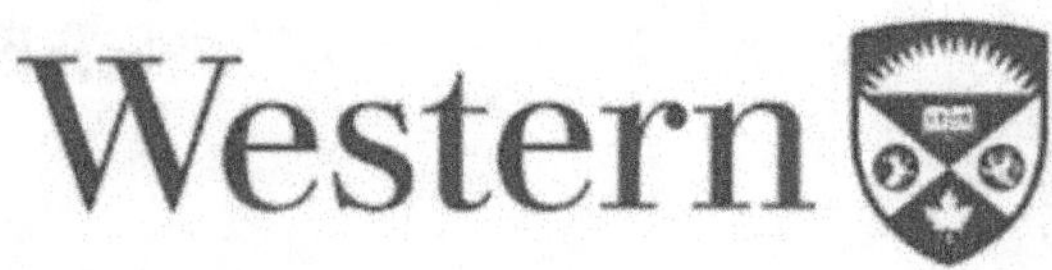

THE WESTERN WAY

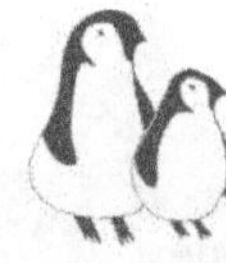

Internal Medicine: Respirology

A.B.R Thomson

Table of Contents

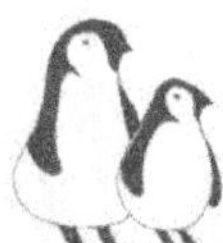

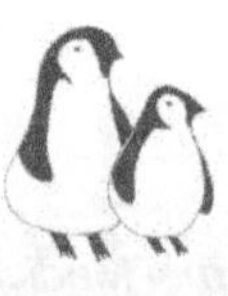

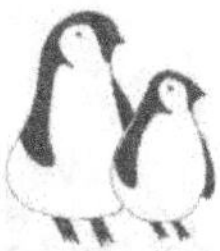

DISCLAIMER

The primary purpose of this publication is education. The author, editor and publisher acknowledge that the development of new material opens to way for possible errors – what is correct today might not be the standard of care tomorrow. Readers are advised to ensure that the doses of drugs which they use are in compliance with their country's product information, and that the use of any therapeutic agent, be it a pharmaceutical or a technology, should be guided by local guidelines. There is often a wide diversity of professional opinion, and guidelines from one country are not always congruent with another.

The author, editor and publisher do not guarantee the safety, reliability, accuracy, completeness or usefulness of this material.

They disclaim any and all liability for damage and claims that may result from the use of information, publications, technologies, products, and for series provided in this publication.

We have made every attempt to trace the holders of copyright for material reproduced in this book. If by some oversight we have omitted a copyright holder, please contact us.

Thank you

Alan Thomson

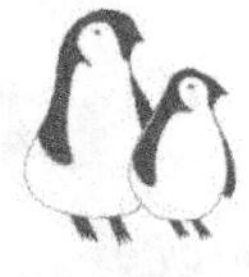

MASTERING THE BOARDS AND THE CANMED OBJECTIVES

Medical Expert

The discussion of complex cases provides the participants with an opportunity to comment on additional focused history and physical examination. They would provide a complete and organized assessment. Participants are encouraged to identify key features, and they develop an approach to problem-solving.

The case discussions, as well as the discussion of cases around a diagnostic imaging, pathological or endoscopic base provides the means for the candidate to establish an appropriate management plan based on the best available evidence to clinical practice. Throughout, an attempt is made to develop strategies for diagnosis and development of clinical reasoning skills.

Communicator

The participants demonstrate their ability to communicate their knowledge, clinical findings, and management plan in a respectful, concise and interactive manner. When the participants play the role of examiners, they demonstrate their ability to listen actively and effectively, to ask questions in an open-ended manner, and to provide constructive, helpful feedback in a professional and non-intimidating manner.

Collaborator

The participants use the "you have a green consult card" technique of answering questions as fast as they are able, and then to interact with another health professional participant to move forward the discussion and problem solving. This helps the participants to build upon what they have already learned about the importance of collegial interaction.

Manager

The participants are provided with assignments in advance of the three day GI Practice Review. There is much work for them to complete before as well as afterwards, so they learn to manage their time effectively, and to complete the assigned tasks proficiently and on time. They learn to work in teams to achieve answers from small group participation, and then to share this with other small group participants through effective delegation of work. Some of the material they must access demands that they use information technology effectively to access information that will help to facilitate the delineation of adequately broad differential diagnoses, as well as rational and cost effective management plans.

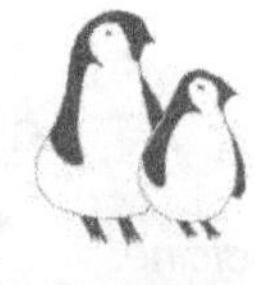

Health Advocate
In the answering of the questions and case discussions, the participants are required to consider the risks, benefits, and costs and impacts of investigations and therapeutic alliances upon the patient and their loved ones.

Scholar
By committing to the pre and post-study requirements, plus the intense three day active learning Practice Review with colleagues is a demonstration of commitment to personal education. Through the interactive nature of the discussions and the use of the "green consult card", they reinforce their previous learning of the importance of collaborating and helping one another to learn.

Professional
The participants are coached on how to interact verbally in a professional setting, being straightforward, clear and helpful. They learn to be honest when they cannot answer questions, make a diagnosis, or advance a management plan. They learn how to deal with aggressive or demotivated colleagues, how to deal with knowledge deficits, how to speculate on a missing knowledge byte by using first principals and deductive reasoning. In a safe and supportive setting they learn to seek and accept advice, to acknowledge awareness of personal limitations, and to give and take 360° feedback.

Knowledge
The basic science aspects of gastroenterology are considered in adequate detail to understand the mechanisms of disease, and the basis of investigations and treatment. In this way, the participants respect the importance of an adequate foundation in basic sciences, the designing of clinical research studies to provide an evidence-based approach, the relevance of their management plans being patient-focused, and the need to add "compassionate" to the Three C's of Medical Practice: competent, caring and compassionate.

"They may forget what you said, but they will never forget how you made them feel."

Carl W. Buechner, on teaching.

"With competence, care for the patient. With compassion, care about the person."

Alan B. R. Thomson, on being a physician.

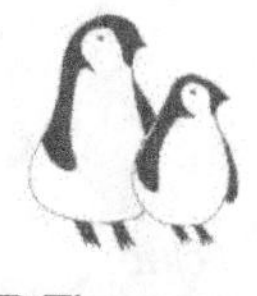

Internal Medicine: *Respirology*
A.B.R Thomson

PROLOGUE

HREs, better known as, High Risk Examinations. After what is often two decades of study, sacrifice, long hours, dedication, ambition and drive, we who have chosen Internal Medicine, and possibly through this a subspecialty, have a HRE, the [Boards] Royal College Examinations. We have been evaluated almost daily by the sadly subjective preceptor based assessments, and now we face the fierce, competitive, winner-take-all objective testing through multiple choice questions (MCQs), and for some the equally challenging OSCE, the objective standardized clinical examination. Well we know that in the real life of providing competent, caring and compassionate care as physicians, as internists, that a patient is neither a MCQ or an OSCE. These examinations are to be passed, a process with which we may not necessarily agree. Yet this is the game in which we have thus far invested over half of our youthful lives. So let us know the rules, follow the rules, work with the rules, and succeed. So that we may move on to do what we have been trained to do, do what we may long to do, care for our patients.

The process by which we study for clinical examinations is so different than for the MCQs: not trivia, but an approach to the big picture, with thoughtful and reasoned deduction towards a diagnosis. Not looking for the answer before us, but understanding the subtle aspects of the directed history and focused physical examination, yielding an informed series of hypotheses, a differential diagnosis to direct investigations of the highly sophisticated laboratory and imaging procedures now available to those who can wait, or pay.

This book provides clinically relevant questions of the process of taking a history and performing a physical examination, with sections on useful background, and where available, evidence-based performance characteristics of the rendering of our clinical skills. Just for fun are included "So you want to be a such-and-such specialist!" to remind us that one if the greatest strengths we can possess to survive in these times, is to smile and even to laugh at ourselves.

Sincerely,

Alan Thomson
Emeritus Distinguished University Professor, University of Alberta
Adjunct Professor, Western University

DEDICATION

To My Family

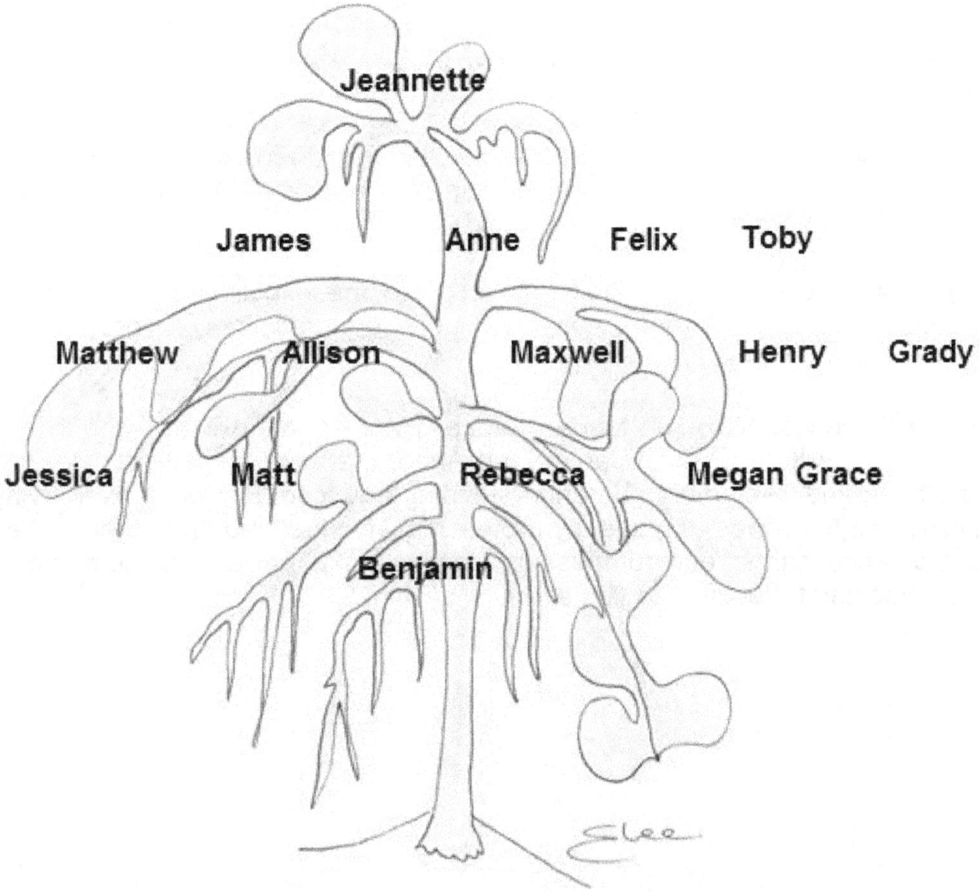

Jeannette

James **Anne** **Felix** **Toby**

Matthew **Allison** **Maxwell** **Henry** **Grady**

Jessica **Matt** **Rebecca** **Megan Grace**

Benjamin

For your support, caring and love

During these challenging years

And always.

Mark 15:34

Luke 23:34

Domenichino 16:41

Corinthians 1:13

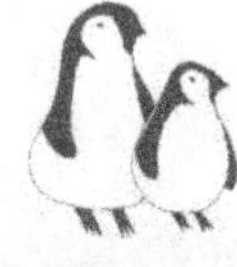

ACKNOWLEDGEMENTS

Patience and patients go hand in hand. So also does the interlocking of young and old, love and justice, equality and fairness. No author can have thoughts transformed into words, no teacher can make ideas become behaviour and wisdom and art, without those special people who turn our minds to the practical – of getting the job done!

Thank you, Naiyana and Duen for translating those terrible scribbles, called my handwriting, into the still magical legibility of the electronic age. Thank you, Sarah, for your creativity and hard work.

My most sincere and heartfelt thanks go to the excellent persons at JP Consulting, and CapStone Academic Publishers. Jessica, you are brilliant, dedicated and caring. Thank you.

When Rebecca, Maxwell, Megan Grace, Henry and Felix ask about their Grandad, I will depend on James and Anne, Matthew and Allison, Jessica and Matt, and Benjamin to be understanding and kind. For what I was trying to say and to do was to make my professional life focused on the three C's - competence, caring, and compassion – and to make my very private personal life dedicated to family – to you all.

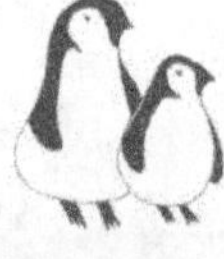

ARE YOU PREPARING FOR EXAMS IN GASTROENTEROLOGY AND HEPATOLOGY?

See the full range of examination preparation and review publications from CAPstone on Amazon.com

Gastroenterology and Hepatology

- First Principles of Gastroenterology and Hepatology in Adults and Children - Volume I – Gastroenterology (ISBN: 978-1494345624)
- First Principles of Gastroenterology and Hepatology in Adults and Children - Volume II - Hepatology and Paediatrics (ISBN: 978-1494345501)
- Medical Mini Review Series in Gastroenterology and Hepatology: Efficient Refresher for the Busy Clinical Gastroenterologist (ISBN: 978-1502472199)
- Medical Mini Review Series in Gastroenterology and Hepatology: Efficient Refresher for the Busy Clinical Gastroenterologist (ISBN: 978-1502472199)
- Practice Review in Gastroenterology (ISBN: 978-1500855321)
- Practice Review in Hepatopancreatobiliary Diseases and Nutrition (ISBN: 978-1500855734)
- Endoscopy and Diagnostic Imaging - Part I: Skin, Nail and Mouth Changes in GI Disease; Esophagus; Stomach; Small intestine; Pancreas (ISBN: 978-1477400579)
- Endoscopy and Diagnostic Imaging - Part II: Colon and Hepatobiliary (ISBN: 978-1477400654)
- Scientific Basis for Clinical Practice in Gastroenterology and Hepatology (ISBN: 978-1475226645)
- The Physiology and Pathophysiology of Gastrointestinal and Hepatopancreaticobiliary Disorders: Preparing for Professional Competence. (ISBN: 978-1500298265)

General Internal Medicine

- Achieving Excellence in the OSCE - Part One: Cardiology to Nephrology (ISBN: 978-1475283037)
- Achieving Excellence in the OSCE - Part Two: Neurology to Rheumatolgy (ISBN: 978-1475276978)
- Mastering the Boards and Clinical Examinations in Internal Medicine, Part I: Cardiology, Endocrinology, Gastroenterology, Hepatology and Nephrology (ISBN: 978-1461024842)
- Mastering The Boards and Clinical Examinations In Internal Medicine, part II: Neurology, Respirology and Rheumatology (ISBN: 978-1478392736)
- Bits and Bytes: Surviving Morning Rounds (ISBN: 978-1478295365)

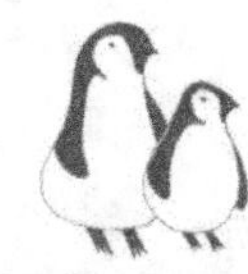

RESPIROLOGY

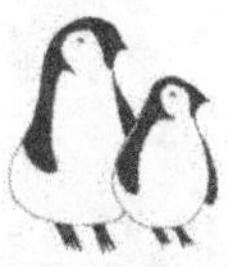

COMMONLY USED TERMS

- Pectus carinatum
  - Pigeon chest
- Pectus excavatum
  - Funnel test
- Adventitial sounds
  - Continuous "wheezes"
  - Discontinuous "crackles"
- Inspiratory wheeze
  - Severe airway narrowing
- Stridor
  - Foreign body tumour
    - Gas inhalation
    - Anaphylaxis
    - Epiglottitis
    - Bilateral vocal cord palsy
- Bronchial breath sounds
  - Normal
  - Pneumonia
  - Fibrosis
  - Effusion
  - Collapse
- Broadbent sign
  - Systolic retraction of intercostals space, especially seen at the post auxiliary line just below the angle of the scapula, with cardiac hypertrophy or fibrous pericarditis
- Pulsus alternans
  - Strong/weak pulse in heart failure
- Sinus arrhythmia
  - ↑HR with inspiration
- Pulsus paradoxicus
  - The normal ↑height of pulse wave with inspiration is lost
- Krönig isthmus
  - A posterior band of resonance 2 inches wide across the shoulder from the apex of the lung, which extends 1 inch above the clavicles
- Distinguish pulmonary rub versus rales
  - Present in both phases of respiration, but rub is enhanced by increasing the pressure on the stethoscope (closer to ear), and a rub is not affected by coughing
- Pectoriloquy
  - ↑ Intensity of spoken voice
  - Bronchophony - ↑clarity of the spoken voice

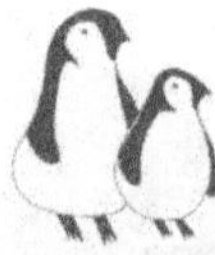

- Pursed-lip breathing
  - Pursed lips increase positive pressure in the weakened bronchial airways in emphysema and COPD, thereby helping to prevent the airway trapping
- Kussmaul breathing
  - Rapid, deep breathing due to metabolic-diabetic ketoacidosis, lactic acidosis, uremia
  - Drugs and poisons – methanol, ethylene glycol, ASA, paraldehyde
- When orthopnea is due to lung disease
  - Dyspnea relieved by sitting up is usually due to L-CHF, but may rarely occur with bilateral bullous apical disease, when sitting up improves the ventilation/perfusion matching and gas exchange in the normal lower lung
- Horner syndrome – apical lung tumour compressing sympathetic nerves in neck, causing myosis, ptosis and anhydrosis

- What are you looking for when you are examining accessory muscles?
  - Motion in scalene muscles (earliest affected), sternocleidomastoid muscles, neck muscles, in drawing of intercostal spaces and supraclavicular fossa
  - Abdominal motion when person inspires
- What paradoxical respiration is
  - The abdomen draws inward on inspiration when it normally should move outward due to diaphragm descent
- Position of trachea
  - Palpate the trachea in the suprasternal notch to determine if it is midline
  - Trachea is deviated to *ipsilateral* side in atelectasis, fibrosis, lung collapse

- Give an approach to the auscultation of the breath sounds to determine the nature of underlying lung disease.

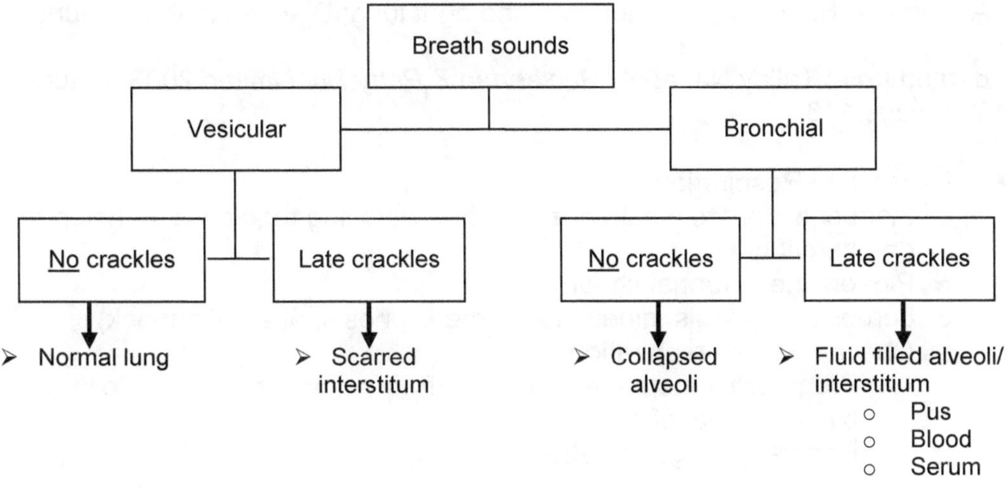

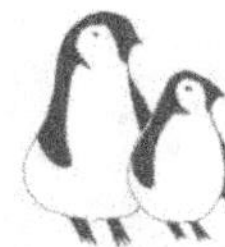

CHEST EXAMINATION

➢ Inspection

Surface anatomy for underlying lobes of the lung.

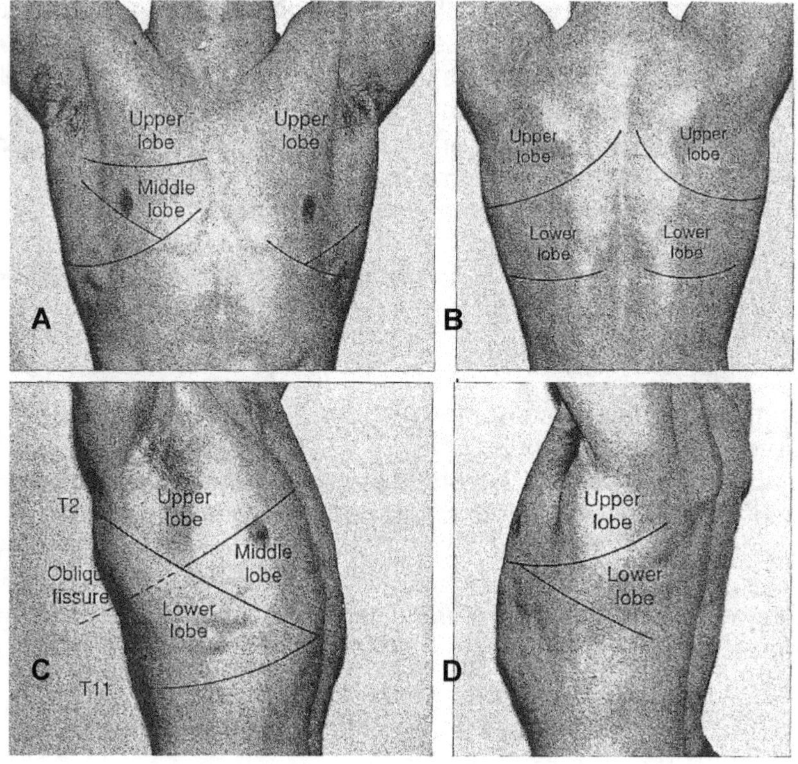

A, anterior; B, posterior; C, lobes of the right lung; D, lobes of the left lung.

Adapted from: Talley NJ, et al. *Maclennan & Petty Pty Limited* 2003, Figure 4.7.2, page 116.

- Patterns of Respiration
  - Instruct patient to inhale deeply while watching for slow expansion of one hemithorax
  - Pigeon chest, funnel chest
  - Lordosis, kyphosis, gibbus (extreme kyphosis, aka hunchback)
  - Cheyne-Stokes respiration
    - Progressive increase in depth $\pm$ frequency of breathing, followed by an interval of apnea
    - Regularly irregular pattern

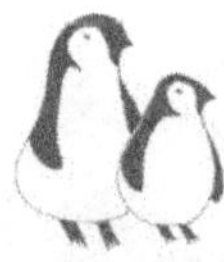

- o Biot breathing
  - A series of increase in the depth ± frequency of breathing, followed by an interval of apnea, without the Cheyne-Stokes regular-irregular pattern

➢ Abnormalities in rhythm of respiration.
- o Abnormal rhythms of respiration usually result from lesions in the neurogenic control of the respiratory pump.
- o They help to localize the site of neurologic lesions. Abnormalities of respiratory rhythm are found in the following sequence from the uppermost to the lower-most neurologic centre.
  - Cheyne-Stokes respiration
  - Biot's respiration
  - Apneustic breathing
  - Central hyperventilation
  - Ataxic (agonal) respiration

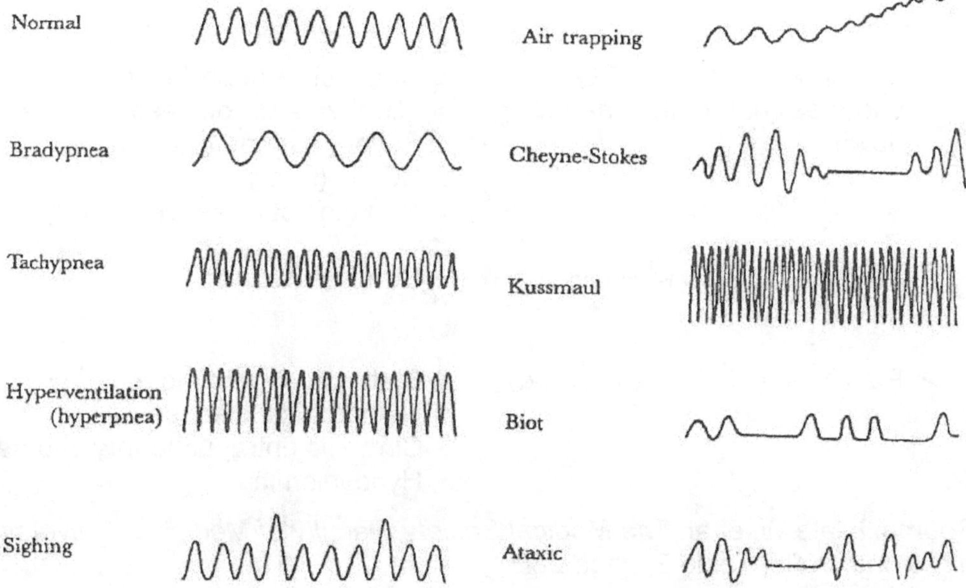

Adapted from: Mangione S. *Hanley & Belfus* 2000, page 279.

- Perform a focused physical examination for causes of Cheyne-Stokes respiration.

  - o All causes of heart failure
  - o Renal failure
  - o ↑ intracranial pressure

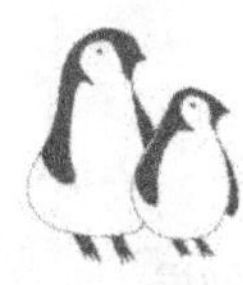

Chest Asymmetry

- Causes
  - Atelectasis
  - Pleural effusion
  - Severe pneumonia
- Complications
  - Cyanosis, chibbing
  - Asterixis (hypercapnea)

Adapted from: Mangione S. *Hanley & Belfus*, 2000, pages 281 and 282.

- Dyspnea, position

- Causes

Useful background: Types of positional dyspnea

Type	Possible Causes
Orthopnea (dyspnea (SOB, shortness of breath) when lying down	Congestive heart failure Mitral valvular disease Severe asthma (rarely) COPD (rarely) Neurological diseases (rarely)
Trepopnea (SOB when lying on one side)	Congestive heart failure
Platypnea (SOB when seated)	Status post pneumonectomy Neurological diseases Cirrhosis (intrapulmonary shunts) Hypovolemia

Source: Filate W, et al. *The Medical Society, Faculty of Medicine, University of Toronto* 2005, Table 2, page 282.

- Little trick

- Orthopnea
  - Dyspnea at rest
  - Unusual in lung disease, or severe anemia

- Tachypnea (↑ rate of breathing, >20/min)
  - If present – suggests cardiopulmonary disease (CPD)
  - If absent – argues strongly against CPD

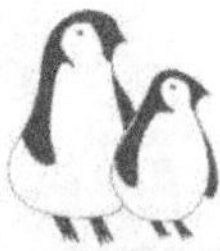

- Hyperpnea (increase rate and depth [tidal volume] of breathing)
  - Finding in anion-gap metabolic acidosis ("**MAKE UP** a **L**ist")

Methanol	**U**remia
Aspirin	**P**araldehyde
Ketoacidosis	
Ethylene Glycol ingested	**L**actoacidosis

Source: Mangione S. *Hanley & Belfus* 2000, pages 278 to 280.

SO YOU WANT TO BE A RESPIROLOGIST!

- Give the Behcet syndrome.
  - Aphthous ulcers in mouth and genitals, associated with arthritis, uvertis and various neurological disorders

Source: Mangione S. *Hanley & Belfus* 2000, page 67.

➢ Palpation
  - Chest wall ~ 3 to 5 cm
  - Hemidiaphragm ~ 1 cm

SO YOU WANT TO BE A RESPIROLOGIST!

- Does pneumonia increase or decrease tactile vocal fremitus (TVF)?
  - ↓ TVF in bronchopneumonia (involving bronchial alveolar pneumonia (fluid in the alveoli plus air in the bronchi)

Source: Mangione S*Hanley & Belfus*, 2000, page 288.

➢ Tactile vocal fremitus (TVF)

Transmission	Possible Pathologies
○ Increased	– Consolidation (e.g., pneumonia)
○ Decreased	
– Unilateral	▪ Atelectasis, bronchial obstruction, pleural effusion, pneumothorax, pleura thickening
– Bilateral	▪ Chest wall thickening (muscle, fat), COPD, Bilateral pleural effusion

- Perform a focused physical examination to distinguish between peripheral versus **central cyanosis**.

	Peripheral	Central
○ Site	Hands, feet*	Lips
○ Temperature	Cold	warm
○ Clubbing	-	+
○ Effect of cold	Worse	No change
○ pO2	Normal	↓
○ pCO2	Normal, or ↓	↑
○ Polycythemia	Yes	No

*Note: lips may be affected in persons with peripheral cyanosis, but the warm breath will reduce this cyanosis.

➢ Auscultation: Breath Sounds

○ Normal auscultatory breath sounds

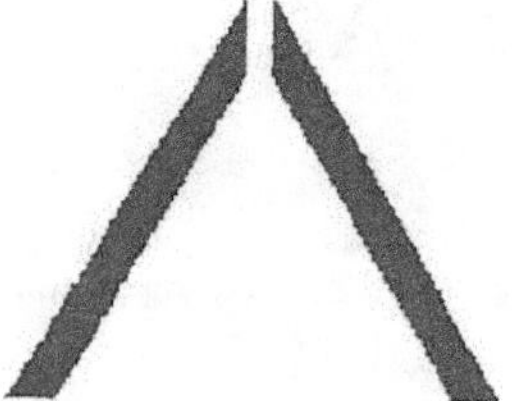

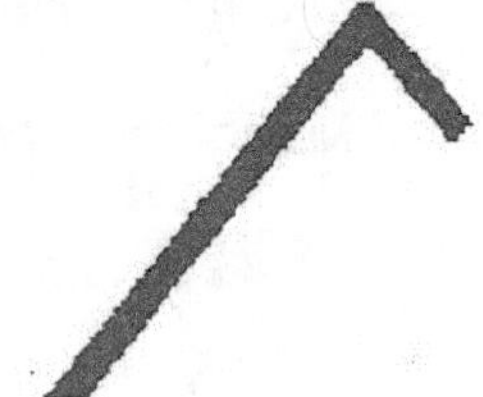

Tubular (tracheal/bronchial) Bronchovesicular Vesicular (soft/muffled)

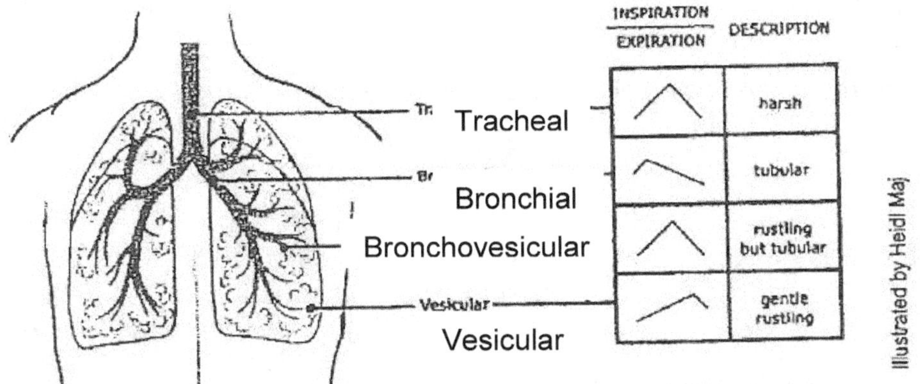

Adapted from: Filate W, et al. *The Medical Society, Faculty of Medicine, University of Toronto* 2005, Figure 4, page 286.

Respiratory Sound	Mechanisms	Origin	Acoustics	Relevance
○ Normal lung sound	- Turbulent flow vortices	- Central airways (expiration), lobar to segmental airway (inspiration)	- Low-pass filtered noise (range < 100 to 1,000 Hz)	- Regional ventilation, airway caliber
○ Normal tracheal sound	- Turbulent flow, flow impinging on airway walls	- Pharynx, larynx, trachea, large airways	- Noise with resonances (range < 100 to > 3,000 Hz)	- Upper airway configuration

- Abnormal breath sounds

Characteristic	Tracheal	Bronchial	Bronchovesicular	Vesicular
○ Description	Harsh	Air rushing through tube	Rustling, but tubular	Gentle rustling
○ Intensity	Very loud	Loud	Moderate	Soft
○ Pitch	Very high	High	Moderate	Low
○ Insp./exp. Ratio	1:1	1:3	1:1	3:1
○ Normal Location	Extrathoracic trachea	Manubrium sterni	Mainstem bronchi	Peripheral lung fields

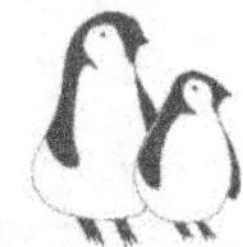

Respiratory Sound	Mechanisms	Origin	Acoustics	Relevance
o Wheeze	- Airway wall flutter (vortex shedding	- Central and lower airways	- Sinusoid (range 100 to > 1,000 Hz; duration, typically > 80 ms)	- Airway obstruction, flow limitation
o Rhonchus	- Rupture of fluid films	- Large airways	- Series of rapidly dampened sinusoids (typically < 300 Hz and duration > 100 ms)	- Secretions, abnormal airway collapsibility
o Crackle	- Airway wall stress-relaxation	- Central and lower airways	- Rapidly dampened wave deflection (duration typically < 20 ms)	- Airway closure, secretions

Adapted from: Mangione S. *Hanley & Belfus* 2000, page 279 and 297;and Filate W., et al. *The Medical Society, Faculty of Medicine, University of Toronto* 2005, Table 6, page 286.

Lung disease	Breath sounds	Adventitious lung sound
o Pneumonia	- Harsh/bronchial or absent	▪ Late inspiratory crackles
o Atelectasis		
o Pneumothorax	- ↓/Absent	▪ None
o Emphysema	- ↓	▪ Early inspiratory crackles
o Chronic bronchitis	- Normal	▪ Wheezes, crackles
o Pulmonary fibrosis	- Harsh	▪ Inspiratory crackles
o Congestive heart failure	- ↓	▪ Inspiratory crackles
o Pleural effusion	- ↓	▪ None
o Asthma	- ↓	▪ Wheezes

Source: Mangione S. *Hanley & Belfus* 2000, page 304.

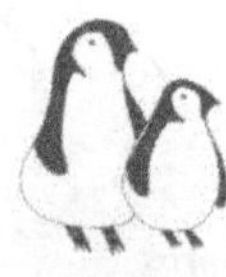

- Give the performance characteristics for pulmonary auscultation for breath sounds and vocal resonance.

Finding	PLR
o Breath sound score	
- Detecting chronic airflow obstruction	
<9	10.2
10-12	3.6
o Diminished breath sounds	
- Detecting underlying pleural effusion in mechanically ventilated patient	4.3
- Detecting asthma during methacholine challenge	4.2
- Detecting pneumonia in patients with cough and fever	2.3
o Bronchial breath sounds	
- Detecting pneumonia in patients with cough and fever	3.3
o Egophony	
- Detecting pneumonia in patients with cough and fever	4.1

Abbreviation: PLR, positive likelihood ratio

Adapted from: McGee SR. *Saunders/Elsevier* 2007, Box 27.1, page 330.

- Give the characteristics of pulmonary crackles in 3 cardiopulmonary disorders.

Diagnosis	Mean number of crackles per inspiration	Timing of crackle	Type of crackle
o Pulmonary fibrosis	6-14	Late inspiratory (0.5→0.9)	Fine
o Pneumonia	3-7	Paninspiratory (0.3→0.7)	Coarse
o Chronic airflow obstruction	1-4	Early inspiratory (0.3→0.5)	Coarse or fine
o Congestive heart failure	4-9	Late or paninspiratory (0.4→0.8)	Coarse or fine

Permission granted: McGee SR. *Saunders/Elsevier* 2007, page 339.

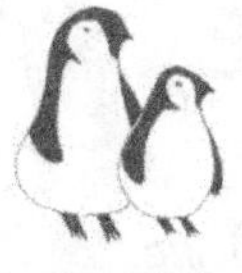

- Give the characteristics of **abnormal breath sounds**.

Recommended ATS Nomenclature	Acoustic Characteristics	Wave Form
o Coarse crackle (aka "coarse rale")	- Discontinuous interrupted explosive sounds - Loud low pitch	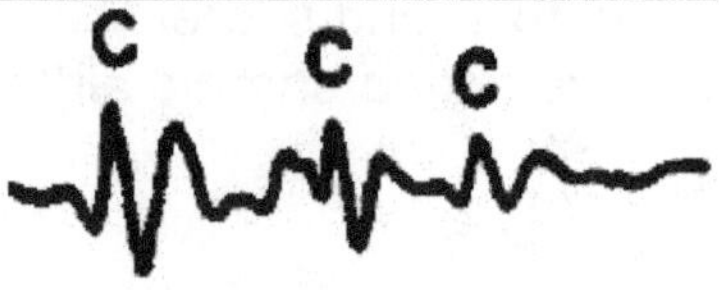
o Fine crackle (aka "fine rale crepitation")	- Discontinuous, interrupted explosive sounds - Less loud than coarse rale, and shorter duration; higher in pitch than coarse rales or crackles	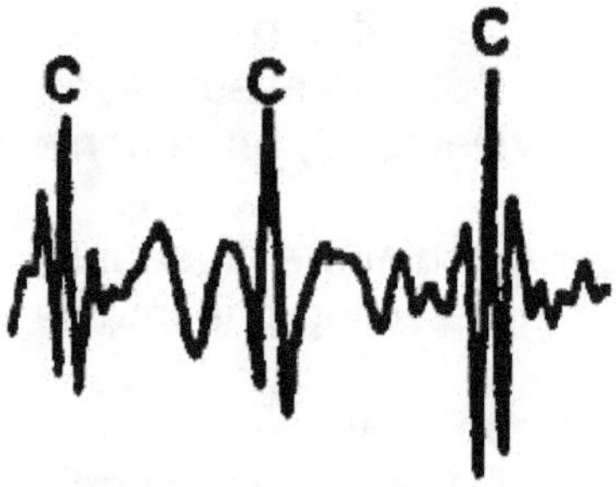
o Wheeze (aka "sibilant rhonchus")	- Continuous sounds - Longer than 250 ms, high pitched	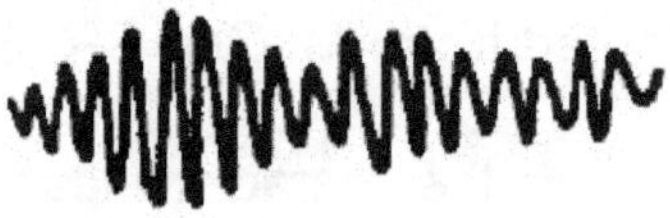
o Rhoncus (aka "sonorous rhonchus")	- Continuous sounds - Longer than 250 ms - low pitch - snoring sound	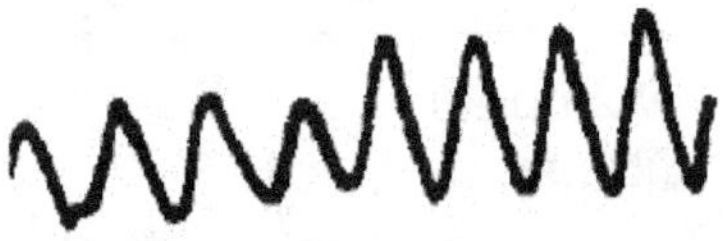

Abbreviation: C, Crackles

Adapted from: Mangione S. *Hanley & Belfus* 2000, page 310.

- Crackles
  - Normal crackles are usually end-inspiratory and high-pitched, and resemble the late inspiratory crackles of interstitial fibrosis.
  - They usually resolve after a few deep inspirations.

- In healthy persons, crackles represent the reinflation of atelectatic lung units. The greater number of collapsed units, the greater the number of crackles generated. These crackles are generally limited to the posterior lung bases. They occur frequently in people who have been breathing close to their functional residual capacity, and then are suddenly asked to take a deep breath. Because a mild degree of basilar collapse is common in healthy persons breathing shallowly below closing capacity, many basilar airways are collapsed. This collapse leads to the reabsorption of oxygen and further atelectasis. The sudden reopening of these airways on inspiration generates the crackles.

Adapted from: Mangione S. *Hanley & Belfus* 2000, page 317.

➢ Cause

- Give the causes of crackles and bronchial breath sounds.
    - Late inspiration crackles (produced by reopening small airways in inspiration):
        - Interstitial fibrosis
            - Interstitial edema
            - Pneumonia
            - Pulmonary hemorrhage
            - CHF
    - Mid inspiration crackles
        - Usually pathogenomic of bronchiectasis
    - Bronchial Breath Sounds
    - Higher and higher-pitch than vesicular breath sounds.
    - Present in areas of airless lungs and patent bronchi (alveolar pneumonia) loading to collapse of alveolar lung tissue, or filling of alveoli with pus, blood or edema fluid, or rarely branchial breath sounds may be heard over areas of severe fibrosis.
    - Chest X-ray may show air bronchogram (air-filled bronchi against the background of disease, airless, consolidated alveoli (lung parenchyma).

Source: Mangione S. *Hanley & Belfus* 2000, page 307.

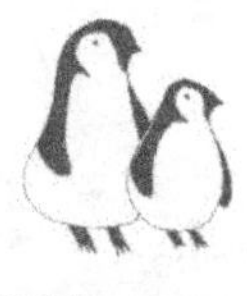

Useful background: Performance characteristics of crackles and wheezes heard on pulmonary auscultation

Finding	PLR
o CRACKLES	
– Detecting pulmonary fibrosis in asbestos workers	5.9
– Detecting elevated left atrial pressure in patients with cardiomyopathy	3.4
– Detecting myocardial infarction in patients with chest pain	2.1
– Detecting pneumonia in patients with cough and fever	1.8
o EARLY INSPIRATORY CRACKLES	
– Detecting chronic airflow obstruction in patients with crackles	14.6
– Detecting severe disease in patients with chronic airflow obstruction	20.8
o UNFORCED WHEEZING	
– Detecting chronic airflow obstruction	2.8
o Wheezing during methacholine challenge testing	
– Detecting asthma	6.0

Abbreviation: PLR, positive likelihood ratio

Crackles from pulmonary edema disappear on coughing, while pleural rub does not. Crackles from fibrosing alveolitis do not disappear on coughing, and lessen on leaning forward.

Adapted from: McGee SR. *Saunders/Elsevier* 2007, Box 27.2, page 338.

Sweet Nothings:

- Posture-induced crackles (PIC) are associated with elevated values of the pulmonary venous compliance. PIC is an independent variable for risk assessment after the number of disease coronary vessels, and increased PCWP (pulmonary capillary wedge pressure).
- A localized persistent rhonchus may indicate underlying lung cancer.

Source: Mangione S. *Hanley & Belfus* 2000, page 323.

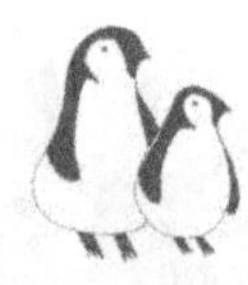

SO YOU WANT TO BE A RESPIROLOGIST!

- Distinguish a pleural rub from a crackle, a wheeze and a pericardial rub.

  - A pleural rub
    - Present during both inspiration and expiration (never present only in expiration)
    - Does not change with coughing
    - Long, louder, lower-pitched than crackle
    - May be palpable

Graphic representation

  - A wheeze
    - Usually occur in expiration only, whereas rubs are usually heard in both inspiration and expiration, or just in inspiration, but never only in expiration.
  - A pericardial rub
    - If the rub persists when the breath is held, then (dah!) it is more likely a pericardial than a pleural rub.

Source: Mangione S. *Hanley & Belfus* 2000, pages 310, 328 and 329.

- How can you suspect if a person's dyspnea is on an hysterical basis?
    - The breathing is deep, and the person holds their breath after about every six breaths.

SO YOU WANT TO BE RESPIROLOGIST!

- Pulmonary crackles are caused by many lung conditions, and finger clubbing is caused by many diseases of lung, heart, GI tract, etc.. But what four pulmonary conditions are associated with both lung crackles and finger clubbing, and what are the characteristics of the crackles which might help to distinguish the cause?
    - Immune – fibrosing alveolitis (crackles-fine)
    - Infiltrative – bronchogenic lung cancer (localized)
    - Infections – bronchiectasis (course)
    - Industrial – asbestosis

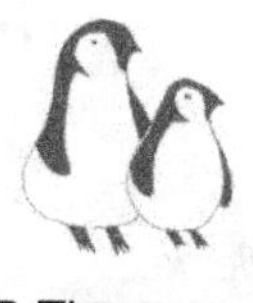

- Give the role of chest examination in the diagnosis of lung disease.

Disease	Trachea	Fremitus	Percussion Note	Breath Sounds	Advential Breath Sounds	Transmitted Breath Sounds
➢ Normal lung	Midline	Normal	Resonant	Vesicular	Late-inspiratory crackles at bases (resolve with deep breaths)	Absent
➢ Consolidation (pneumonia, hemorrhage)	Midline	↑	Dull	Bronchial	Late-inspiratory crackles	+
➢ Pulmonary fibrosis	Midline	Normal ↑	Resonant	Brocnho-vesicular	Late-inspiratory crackles	-
➢ Bronch-iectasis	Midline	Normal	Resonant	Vesicular	Mid-in-spiratory crackles	-
➢ Bronchitis	Midline	Normal	Normal to hyper-resonant	Vesicular	Early-in-spiratory crackles	-
➢ Emphysema	Midline	↓	Hyper-resonant	Diminished vesicular	Usually absent	-
➢ Large pleural effusion	Shifted to opposite side	↓/0	Flat	Bronchial immediately above effusion Absent over effusion	? Rub above effusion	May be present above effusion Absent over effusion
➢ Pneumo-thorax	Shifted to opposite side	↓/0	Tympanic	-	-	-
➢ Atelectasis (patent bronchi)	Shifted to same side	↑	Dull	Bronchial	-	+
➢ Atelectasis (plugged bronchi)	Shifted to same side	↓/0	Dull	-	-	-
➢ Status asthmaticus	Midline	↓	Hyper-resonant	Vesicular	Inspiratory/ expiratory wheezes	-

Abbreviation: advent, adventitial; trans, transmitted

Adapted from: Mangione S. *Hanley & Belfus* 2000, pages 291-292 and 297.

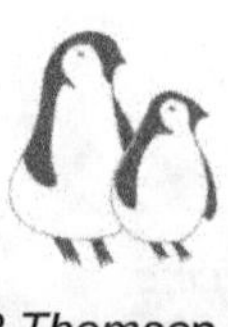

➢ Comparison of the physical findings in the chest for consolidation, collapse, effusion and fibrosis.

	Consolidation	Collapse	Effusion	Fibrosis
o Inspection				
– Chest wall movement	↓	↓	↓	↓ Apical, flattening of chest on the affected side
o Palpation				
– Tactile vocal fremitus (TVF; "E", "1-2-3", "99") (Same as vocal resonance, VR)	↑ alveolar pneumonia (bronchi patent) ↓ broncho-pneumonia	Alveolar ↑ TVF	↑ above effusion; absent over effusion	↓, or absent
o Displaced trachea	-	Towards collapse	Away from effusion	Towards the fibrosis
o Percussion dullness	+	+	*	+
o Auscultation				
– Breath sounds	Bronchial	Broncho-vesicular	Bronchial above fluid, absent over fluid	↓ Bronchial
o Adventitial sounds	Crackles	Crackles	-	Crackles
o Ausculatory vocal resonance (E-E-E, egophony, whispered pectoriloquy, broncho-phony)	One-One-One; Same as TVF	Same as TVF	Same for TVF	Same as TVF

Abbreviations: TVF, tactile vocal fremitus; VR (Ausculatory) vocal resonance.

Adapted from: Talley N. J., et al. *Maclennan & Petty Pty Limited* 2003, Table 4.8, page 123.

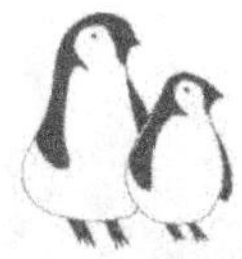

TRACHEAL DEVIATION

➢ Clinical

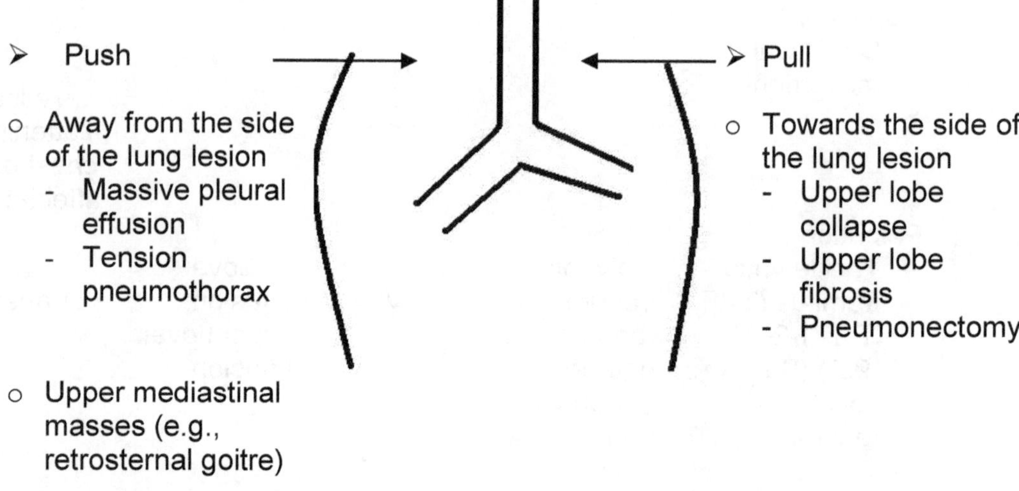

- Perform a directed physical examination of the pulmonary system for tracheal deviation.
    - Lung findings in the affected side
        - ↓tactile vocal fremitus
        - Dullness
        - ↓breath sounds
    - Tracheal deviation to the same side as the above lung findings, which is due to the pull effect of atelectasis
    - Tracheal deviation to the normal side of the lung, due to the push effect of pleural effusion

Adapted from: Talley NJ, et al. *Maclennan & Petty Pty Limited* 2003, Table 4.6, page 110; Mangione S. *Hanley & Belfus* 2000, page 287.

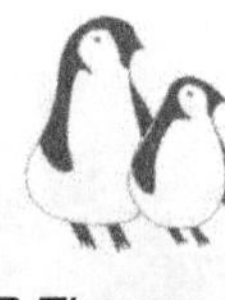

- Percussion

- Give the types of percussion notes and pathological examples of changes.

Percussion note	Pathologic Example
Dullness	- Lobar pneumonia - Pleural effusion - Hemothorax - Empyema - Atelectasis - Tumour
Resonance	- Chronic bronchitis
Hyperresonance	- Emphysema, pneumothorax - Asthma

- Perform a focused physical examination to distinguish between the four commonest causes of dullness at the base of the lung.

	Chest Wall Movement	TVR	Tracheal Deviation	Auscultation
Pleural effusion	↓	↓	+/-	↓ BS
Pleural thickening (fibrosis)	Flattening		Yes	Crackles bronchial breathing
Consolidation (pneumonia)	↓	↑	No	↑ BS bronchial crackles breathing
Collapse (atelectasis)	↓		+	↓ BS

Abbreviation: TVR, tactile vocale resonance; BS, breath sounds

Useful background:

- Mechanisms causing abnormalities in pO2 and pCO2
  - ↓ ventilation - ↑ pCO2
  - ↓ diffusion - ↓ pO2
  - Ventilation/perfusion defects - ↓ pO2, ↓ pCO2
  - ↓ compliance

- Causes of decreased compliance
  - Fibrosis
  - Congestion
  - Deformity of chest wall

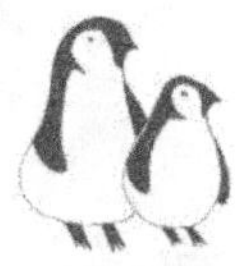

- Acid-base balance: handling of H^+
  - In kidney, H^+ combines with HCO_3^-, NH_3^-, $NaHPO_4$
  - In blood, H^+ is buffered by HCO_3^-, PO_4^{2-} or protein (especially reduced hemoglobin)
  - Acid (H^+) and HCO_3^- ($H^+ + HCO_3^- \rightarrow H_2CO_3$, AKA carbonic acid) shift the oxygen dissociation curve to the right, causing hemoglobin unload its O_2.

SO YOU WANT TO BE A RESPIROLOGIST!

- Are breath sounds reduced when ausculated over a pleural effusion?

  "It depends!"
  - Above the effusion-normal
  - At the margin of the effusion-increased
  - Over the rest of the effusion-reduced

Source: Mangione S. *Hanley & Belfus* 2000, page 305.

- Give the effect of coughing on expiratory crackles.
  - Obstructive disease, decreased course expiratory crackles restrictive disease, no change with coughing.

Source: Mangione S. *Hanley & Belfus* 2000, page 315.

- Are late inspiratory crackles common in all types of intestinal lung disease?
  - Common in Ideaoathic Pulmonary Fibrosis (IPF) or Asbestosis (60%), but uncommon in sarcoidosis (18%; upper lobe and peribronchial fibrosis, vs lower lobe and subpleural fibrosis in IPF).

Source: Mangione S.*Hanley & Belfus* 2000, page 317.

- Give is the cause of a clicking sound which is synchronous with systole.
  - Left-side pneumothorax

- How does "Biot breathing" differ from Cheyne-Stokes breathing?
  - Short periods of irregular breathing (varying rate and depth), Followed by periods of apnea
  - Usually seen in association with meningitis
  - Biot breathing lacks the waxing and waning of Cheyne-Stokes breathing

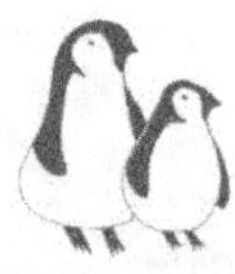

SO YOU WANT TO BE A RESPIROLOGIST!

- Give the meaning of respiratory alternans (aka paradoxical respiration, or abdominal paradox?

  - Normally with inspiration both chest and abdominal wall rises. With muscular weakness and fatigue, the abdominal wall does not rise.

- In the persons with smoker's face and nicotine staining of fingers, pursed lips and using the accessory muscles of expiration (intercostals muscles), give the meaning of Dahl's sign.

  - Patches of hyperpigmented cullses above both knees from chronic pressure of the elbows on the skin of the legs resulting from sitting up and leaning forward to breath better (orthopnea), placing the elbows near the knees and fixing the position of the shoulder and the neck muscles to improve the contractility of the accessory muscles and improving basilar perfusion and lung mechanics.

  Source: Mangione S. *Hanley & Belfus* 2000, pages 277 and 280.

- Give the cause of bronchopneumonia in which bronchial breathing as well as other physical findings are usually absent, or minimal.
  - Viral bronchopneumonia

- From inspection of the patient, give how you can distinguish between cyanosis and met-/ sulphemoglobinemia.
  - Usually seen in association with meningitis
  - Persons with an excess of these abnormal hemoglobins do not have dyspnea.

- Give the way in which you can estimate the value of FEV_1/FVC with your stethoscope?

  - Auscultate over sternal notch and time how long it takes the patient to take a deep breath and blow out hard. This gives the forced-expiratory time (FET_0).

FET_0	FEV_1/FVC
>6 sec	$\leq$ 40%
<5 sec	> 60%

Source: Mangione S. *Hanley & Belfus* 2000, page 304.

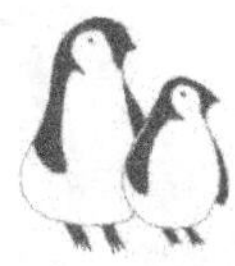

COUGH

➢ Description of "Cough"

Cough		Some Causes
○ Sound		
-	Dry, hacking	▪ Viral interstitial lung disease, ▪ Tumour ▪ Allergies, ▪ Anxiety
-	Chronic, productive	▪ COPD ▪ Bronchiectasis ▪ Abscess ▪ Pneumonia ▪ TB
-	Wheezing	▪ Bronchospasm (Asthma, Allergies) ▪ Congestive heart failure
-	Barking	▪ Epiglottal disease (e.g., "croup")
-	Stridor	▪ Tracheal obstruction
○ Timing		
-	Morning	▪ Smoking
-	Nocturnal	▪ Post-nasal drip ▪ Congestive heart failure ▪ Asthma
-	Upon eating/ drinking	▪ Neuromuscular disease of the upper esophagus (aspiration)

Adapted from: Filate W. et al. *The Medical Society, Faculty of Medicine, University of Toronto* 2005, Table 1, page 281.

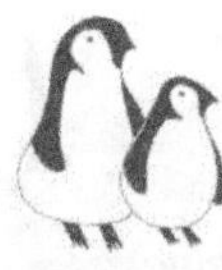

➢ Features of Chronic Cough: Common Causes, Clinical Features and Investigations

Common Causes	Clinical Features
o Upper airway cough syndrome	- Post-nasal drainage - Cobblestoning and mucus in oropharynx - Nasal discharge - Throat clearing
o Cough variant asthma	- Typical features of asthma, such as wheezing, often symptoms
o ACE inhibitor	- Dry, non-productive cough - Onset hours-months - No predisposing factors - Class effect of ACE inhibitors
o Nonasthmatic eosinophilic bronchitis	- Often prolonged in postinfectious setting

Abbreviations: ACE, angiotensin converting enzyme; GI, gastrointestinal

Reproduced with permission: Therapeutics Choices. Sixth Edition. Ottawa, Canada: *Canadian Pharmacist Association* 2012, Table 1, page 633.

➢ Clinical

- Take a directed history for cough.
    - o Cough
        - Acute/chronic (duration)
        - Change
        - Frequency
        - Onset/offset
        - Dry or wet
        - Sputum
            - ▪ Onset/duration
            - ▪ Frequency
            - ▪ Progression
            - ▪ Quantity
            - ▪ Colour
            - ▪ Consistency
            - ▪ Odour

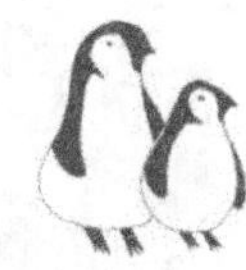

- Hemoptysis
- Mucoid (uninfected) sputum is odourless, transparent, and whitish-gray; small volumes suggest presence of asthma.
- Purulent (infected) sputum contains pus, is often coloured, and large daily volume (50-1000 cc's) suggests bronchiectasis
- Foul-smelling sputum is suggestive of a lung abscess

- Complications
  - Fever, chills
  - Anorexia, weight loss
  - Pleuritic chest pain
  - On/off
  - Dyspnea (SOB), dyspnea on exertion, (SOBOE), paroxysmal nocturnal dyspnea (PND)

- Causes
  - Smoking (pack years)
  - Lung cancer in family
  - Inhalation work
  - TB exposure
  - Travel
  - Sexual orientation
  - Allergies
  - Drugs
  - COPD, CF, asthma
  - CHF, MI, AF
  - Puffers, Rx
  - Sleep
  - Past history
  - Co-morbid illness (CaL, CF, CRF, cirrhosis)

Abbreviations: AF, atrial fibrillation; CaL, cancer of lung; CF, Cystic fibrosis; CHF, congestive heart failure; MI, myocardial infarctions; CRF, chronic renal failure; COPD, chronic obstructive pulmonary disease; PND, paroxysmal nocturnal dyspnea; Rx, medications; SOB, shortness of breath; SOBOE, shortness of breath on exertion.

Adapted from: Jugovic PJ, et al. *Saunders/ Elsevier* 2004, page 124: Filate W, et al. *The Medical Society, Faculty of Medicine, University of Toronto* 2005, page 281.

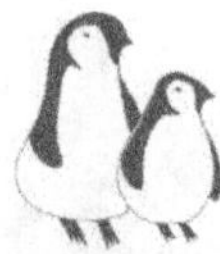

- Sputum
  - Onset/duration, frequency, progression, quantity, colour, consistency, odour, hemoptysis
  - Mucoid (uninfected) sputum
    - Odourless, transparent, and whitish-gray
  - Purulent (infected) sputum
    - Contains pus, and is often coloured
  - Foul-smelling sputum is
    - Suggestive of a lung abscess

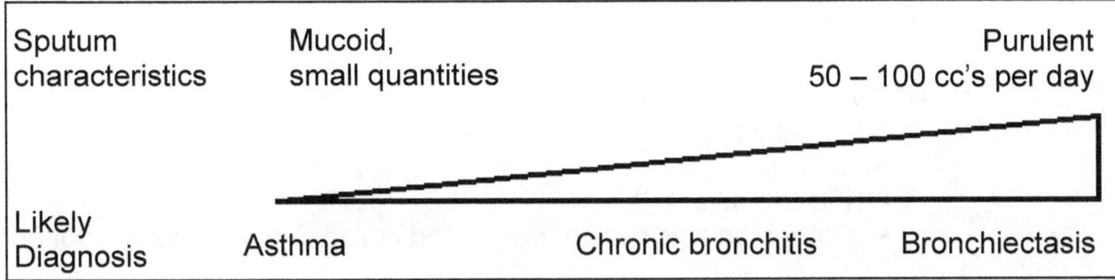

Adapted from: Filate W., et al. *The Medical Society, Faculty of Medicine, University of Toronto* 2005, page 281.

HEMOPTYSIS

- Clinical

- Take a directed history of hemoptysis.
  - Nose
    - Bleeding
  - GI
    - Upper GI bleeding
  - CVS
    - Acute L-CHF, severe mitral stenosis
  - Bleeding diathesis

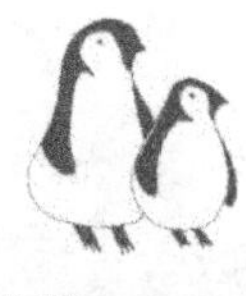

- Respiratory
  - Infection – bronchitis, bronchiectasis, pneumonia, abscess, TB
  - Infarction
  - Infiltration
  - Ischemia – ruptured blood vessel from coughing; Goodpasture's syndrome
  - Cystic fibrosis
  - Foreign body

Abbreviation: L-CHF, left-sided congestive heart failure

Adapted from Talley NJ, et al. *Maclennan & Petty Pty Limited* 2003, Table 4.2, page 101.

➢ Remember

- Rales
  - ↑ by coughing
  - Arise from
    - Fluid in alveoli
    - Bronchiectasis due to associated collapse and/or consolidation

- Increased vocal resonance (VR)
  - Consolidation
  - Cavitation

• Perform a directed physical examination of the pulmonary system for consolidation, collapse, effusion, or fibrosis.

- General inspection
  - Contents of sputum cup (blood, pus etc..)
  - Type of cough
  - Rate and depth of respiration, and breathing pattern at rest and after exercise
  - Accessory muscles of respiration
  - Cheyne-Stokes breathing
  - Kussmaul hyperventilation
  - Temperature chart
  - Anemia
  - Obesity (sleep apnea)
  - Weight loss
  - Wasting, infraclavicular region
  - Mental status change (especially in the elderly)

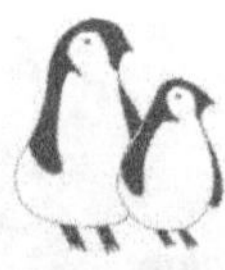

- Face
    - Eyes – Horner syndrome (apical lung cancer)
    - Mouth – central cyanosis of tongue
    - Voice – hoarseness (recurrent laryngeal nerve palsy)
    - Skin – pallor

- Neck
    - Nodes
    - Thyromegaly
    - Trachea
    - Jugular venous pressure (CCF, SVC obstruction)
    - Use of accessory muscles

- Trachea shift towards lesion
    - Atelectasis
    - Fibrosis
    - Pneumonectomy

- Hands
    - Nicotine staining (actually from tobacco tar)
    - Clubbing
    - Cyanosis (peripheral)
    - Wasting, weakness – finger abduction and adduction (lung cancer involving the brachial plexus)
    - Wrist tenderness (hypertrophic pulmonary osteoarhtropathy)
    - Pulse (tachycardia; pulsus paradoxus)
    - Flapping tremor (CO_2 retention)
    - Warm palms and rapid bounding pulse (CO_2 retention)

- Chest
    - Inspect
        - Shape of chest and spine
        - Scars
        - Prominent veins (determine direction of flow)
        - Movement of R/L side of chest
        - Barrel-chest shaped
        - Pemberton's sign (SVC obstruction)
        - Radiotherapy marks
    - Palpate
        - Rib tenderness
        - Expansion
        - Position of trachea
        - Tactile vocal fremitus (TVF) ('ninety nine')
        - Pemberton's sign (superior vena cava obstruction)

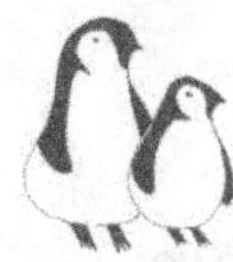

- Percuss
    - Supraclavicular region
    - Dullness or hyperresonance
    - Upper, middle and lower chest on each side, front and back
- Auscultate
    - Breath sounds (vesicular or bronchial)
    - Adventitial sounds (wheeze, crackles, pleural rub; do crackles disappear on coughing? Rub does not).
    - Vocal resonance ("one, one, one"; better than TVF)
    - Murmur of TR
    - Early diastolic Graham Steell murmur
    - P_2, loud ejection click
    - Forced expiratory time (FET, full inspiration to full expiration, over trachea, < 6 seconds is normal)

- Other
    - Breasts
    - Liver
    - Spleen
    - Lower limbs – edema, cyanosis

*Remember to inspect, palpate, percuss, auscultate in right (R). axilla for R. middle lobe disease

Abbreviations: FET, forced expiratory time; SVO, superior vena cava; TR, tricuspid regurgitation; TVF, tactile vocal fremitus

Adapted from: Talley NJ, et al. *Maclennan & Petty Pty Limited* 2003, Figure 4.8, pages 122 and 123.

"There is no achievement without goals."

Robert J. McKaine

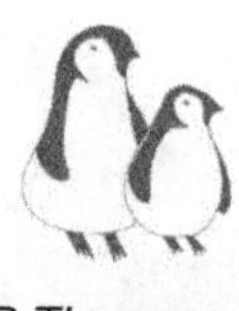

- Clubbing

- Definition
  - Clubbing is a painless focal, usually symmetric enlargement of the connective tissue in the terminal phalanges of the digits of the fingers more than the toes.

- Clinical

- Perform a directed physical examination for the causes of clubbing.

  - CVS
    - Cyanotic congenital heart disease
    - Infective endocarditis
    - Axillary artery aneurysm

  - Lung
    - Lung carcinoma (usually not small cell carcinoma)
    - Bronchial arteriovenous aneurysm
    - Chronic suppuration
      - Bronchiectasis
      - Lung abscess
      - Empyema
    - Idiopathic pulmonary fibrosis
      - Cystic fibrosis
      - Asbestosis
      - Pleural mesothelioma (benign fibrous type) or pleural fibroma

  - Gastrointestinal
    - Cirrhosis
    - Inflammatory bowel disease (Crohn, ulcerative colitis)
    - Celiac disease

  - Endocrine
    - Throtoxicosis
    - Secondary hyperparathyroidism

  - Rare
    - Neurogenic diaphragmatic tumours
    - Pregnancy

  - May be familial or ideopathic

Adapted from: Talley NJ, et al. *Maclennan & Petty Pty Limited* 2003, Table 3.3, page 36.

- Perform a directed physical examination for digital clubbing.

➢ Interphalangeal depth ratio: Measurement of the interphalangeal depth ratio is described in the Figure below. If this ratio exceeds 1, clubbing is present, a conclusion supported by two observations:

  - The interphalangeal depth ratio of normal persons is 0.895 ± 0.041, making the threshold of 1.0 more than 2.5 standard deviations above the normal
  - A ratio of 1.0 distinguishes digits of healthy persons from those of patients with disorders traditionally associated with clubbing (such as cyanotic heart disease and cystic fibrosis). For example, studies demonstrate that 75% to 91% of patients with cystic fibrosis have an interphalangeal depth ratio exceeding 1, but only 0% to 1.5% of normal persons do.
  - A disadvantage to using the hyponychial angle is that special equipment is required for precise measurements.

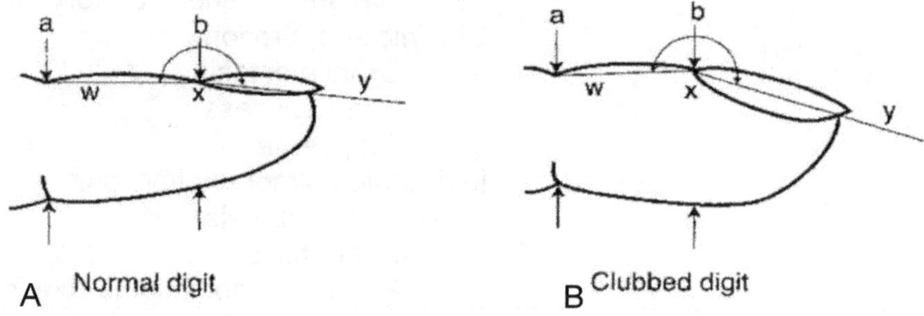

  - A : normal digit
  - B : Clubbed digit
    - The distal interphalangeal joint is denoted by “a”
    - The junction of the nail and skin at the midline is denoted by “b”
    - The interphalangeal depth ratio is the ratio of the digit’s depth measured at “b” divided by that at “a”
    - The hyponychial angle is the angle “wxy”
    - In the Figure, the depth ratio is 0.9 for the normal digit and 1.2 for the clubbed digit (a ratio >1 indicates clubbing) and the hyponychial angle is 185 degrees for the normal digit and 200 degrees for the clubbed digit (a hyponychial angle > 190 degrees indicates clubbing.

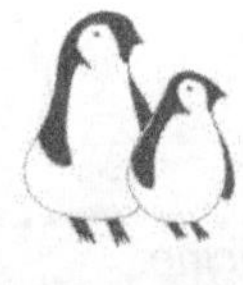

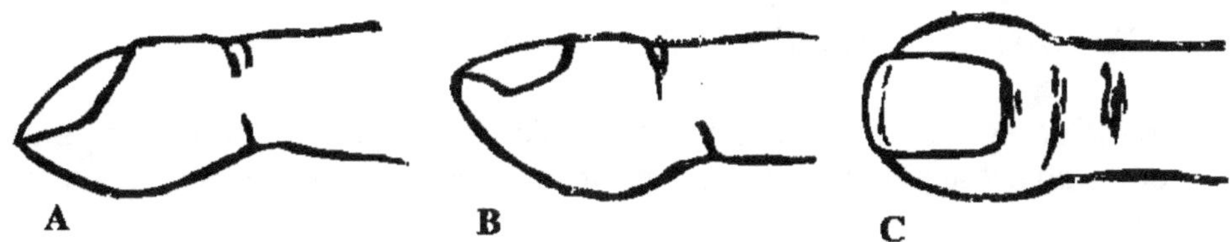

A – Parrot beak-accumulation of connective tissue in proximal portion of distal digit
B – Watchglass-connective tissue at base of nail
C – Drumstick-connective tissue at base of nail

- Schamroth's sign?
  - Disappearance of the diamond-shaped window normally present when the terminal phalanges of paired digits are juxtaposed.

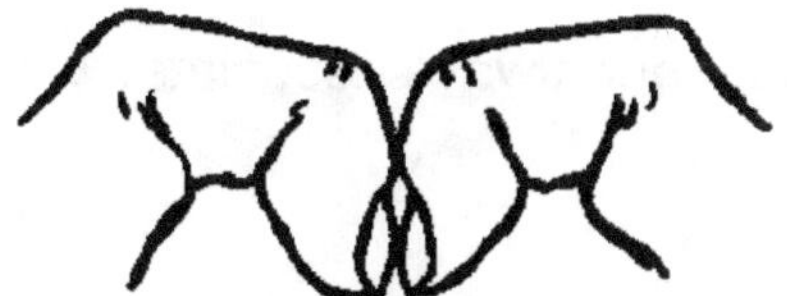

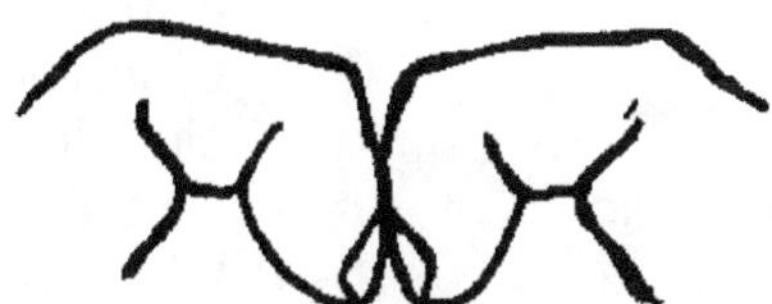

  - Accumulation of connective tissue may occur quickly (<10 days).

Adapted from: Mangione S. *Hanley & Belfus* 2000, pages 482 to 485.

Distinguish between clubbing versus hypertrophic osteoarthropathy.

- Clubbing (sequence of changes)
  - Filling-in of angle between nail and nail bed ("profile sign")
  - ↑ curvature of nail, longitudinal and horizontal
  - Soft tissue swelling of ends of fingers ("drumstick")
  - Nails may be smooth, shiney and brittle

- Hypertrophic osteoarthropathy (bilateral, symmetrical periostitis at ends of bone)
  - Clubbing plus pain and swelling of

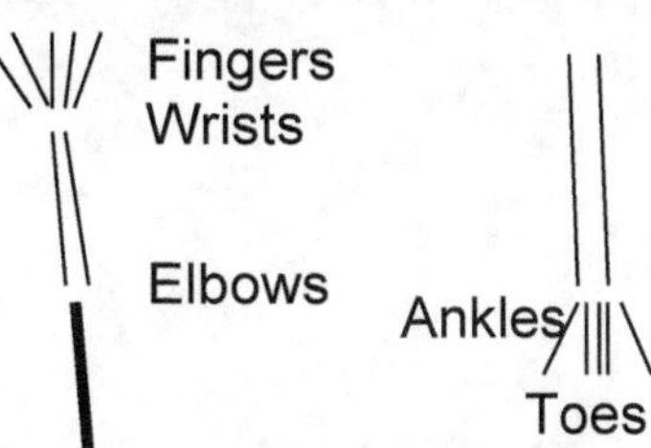

  - Note – clubbing associated with cancer of the lungs (especially peripheral cancer) may be painful

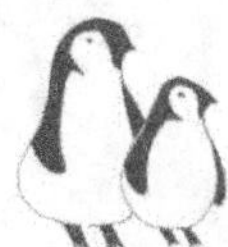

SO YOU WANT TO IMPRESS YOUR STAFF!

- In the context of clubbing and bone pain as well as tenderness, give what other physical signs suggest hypertrophic pulmonary osteoarthropathy (HPO).

  - Pretibial skin
    - Shiny
    - Warm
    - Red
    - Thickened
    - Sweating
  - Hands and feet
    - Sweating
    - Warmth
    - Paresthesias
    - Clubbing, but note: not always associated with clubbing
  - Systemic
    - Sweating
    - Warmth
    - Paresthesias
  - Joints
    - Symmetrical
    - Arthritis-like changes in wrists, elbows, knees, ankles
  - Subcutaneous tissue-coarsening in
    - Hands
    - Feet
    - Face

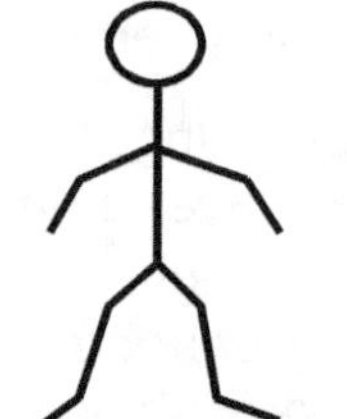

    - Elbows
    - Wrists
    - Knees
    - Ankles
  - Causes
    - Lung
      - Bronchogenic cancer
      - Metastatic lung cancer
      - Mesothelioma
      - Bronchiectasis
      - Lung abscess
      - Chronic empyema
      - Cystic fibrosis - **Note**: HPO almost never occurs with pulmonary interstitial fibrosis
    - CVS
      - Infected aortic bypass graft
    - Liver
      - Cirrhosis
  - Clinical course
    - HPO often resolves with cure of associated condition

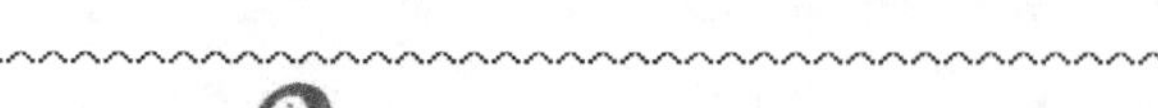

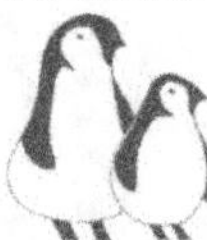

SO YOU WANT TO BE A RESPIROLOGIST!

- Other than from the family history, give how can you distinguish familial from non-familial clubbing.
    - Familial clubbing is
        - Asymmetrical
        - Increases with aging

- Give the cause of unilateral clubbing of the right hand.
    - Aneurysm of the thoracic aorta

- Give the meaning of hypertrophic pulmonary osteoarthropathy.
    - Hypertrophic pulmonary osteoarthropathy is digital clubbing with periostosis (Marie-Bamberger syndrome)
    - A systemic disorder of bones, joints, and soft tissues most commonly associated with an intrathoracic neoplasm (usually bronchogenic carcinoma but also lymphomas and metastatic cancers).
    - Periosteal new-bone proliferation that accompanies digital clubbing, especially prominent in the long bones of the extremities.
    - Other features of symmetric arthritis-like changes in one or more joints (ankles, knees, wrists, and elbows); coarsening of the subcutaneous tissue in the distal portions of arms and legs (and occasionally the face); neurovascular changes in hands and feet (with chronic erythema, paresthesias, and increased sweating).
    - Associations may be seen in
        - Cystic fibrosis,
        - Brochiectasis,
        - Chronic empyema,
        - Lung abscesses (all typically associated with clubbing),
        - Pulmonary interstitial fibrosis

Source: Mangione S. *Hanley & Belfus* 2000, page 485.

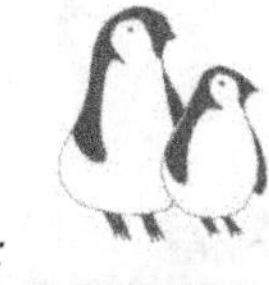

SO YOU WANT TO BE A RESPIROLOGIST!

- Give the condition in which clubbing is associated with pulmonary crackles.
    - Bronchogenic carcinoma (crackles are localized)
    - Bronchiectasis (coarse crackles)
    - Asbestosis
    - Fibrosing alveolitis (fine, end-expiratory, not disappearing on coughing, but disappear on leaning forward)

Source: Baliga RR. *Saunders/Elsevier* 2007, page 282.

SO YOU WANT TO IMPRESS YOUR STAFF!

- Give the circumstances when clubbing of the digits is painful.
    - When digital clubbing is associated with periostosis, periosteal formation of new bone, and hypertrophy (hypertrophic pulmonary osteoarthropathy, [HPO], aka Marie-Bamberger syndrome)
    - The diagnosis of HPO is may be suspected clinically, but is confirmed by the radiological demonstration of periostosis.

SO YOU WANT TO IMPRESS YOUR STAFF!

- Give the findings on examination of the dorsal portion of the fingers for bulimia.
    - Abrasions, excoriations or calluses
        - Suggest chronic trauma on the fingers against the teeth as the sufferer repeatedly attempts to induce vomiting.

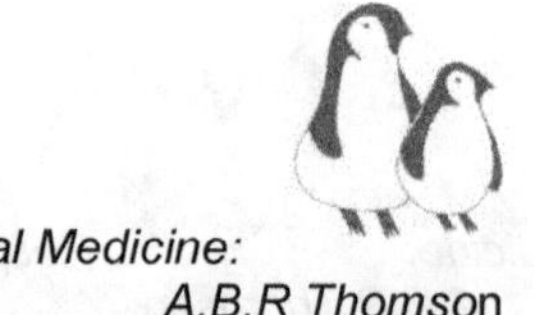

Hypertrophic Osteoarthropathy

Hypertrophic osteoarthropathy is comprised of clubbing of the digits, plus

- Synovia
  - Effusions
- Bones
  - Painful periostosis of long bones
  - Perioteal formation of new bone
- Skin
  - Edema

- There are many causes of clubbing, but give the commonest causes of hypertrophic osteoarthropathy.

  - Lung
    - Cancer
    - Chronic infection (e.g., bronchiectasis)
  - Heart
    - Pulmonary (R)-to-systemic (L) heart shunts

DIAGNOSTIC TESTS FOR PULMONARY DISORDERS

- Function
  - Spirometry
  - Bronchial challenge
  - Lung volumes
  - Diffusion capacity
  - 6-min walk
  - Pulse oximetry
  - Arterial blood gas measurements
  - V / Q scan
- Diagnostic imaging
  - Chest X-ray
  - CT scanning, including angiography
  - Positive emission tomography
  - Bronchoscopy and biopsy
  - Angiography

- Give the diagnostic tests for asthma which are not recommended during pregnancy.

  - Skin testing – not recommended
  - Bronchial challenge testing – contraindicated

- Give the name of 7 pulmonary function tests which are routinely used to assess static lung function, and indicate how these PFTs help in the diagnosis of abstruction to airflow, restrictive lung disease, and impaired gas diffusion.

  - Spirometry
    - Measure
      - FEV1
      - FVC
      - Response of FEV1/FVC to bronchodilators
    - Examples

Finding	Interpretation
FEV1/FVC < 0.7	Airflow obstruction

- ↑ (≥ 12%) in FEV1 or FVC
- ↑ ≥ 200 mL from baseline in FEV1 or FVC
- ↓ FEV1 = ↓ FVC (equal decrease in both FEV1 and FVC
- Note: spirometry may be normal in asthma, and a methacholine bronchoprovacation test is necessary
- Do not improve with bronchodilator
  - COPD

  - Flow-volume loops
    - Scooped-out pattern
      - Improves with bronchodilator
        - Asthma (reversible obstructive airway disease)
        - Tracheal stenosis (fixed obstruction outside the chest)
    - Flattened pattern

  - Lung volume (TLC [total lung capacity], VC [vital capacity], and RV [residual volume])
    - ↓ VC, ↑ RV
      - Airflow obstruction
    - ↓ TLC
      - Restriction lung disease

  - DL_{CO}
    - ↓ DL_{CO}
      - Emphydema
      - Pulmonary fibrosis
      - Bronchiectasis
      - Normal spirometry and lung volumes
      - Pulmonary vascular disease

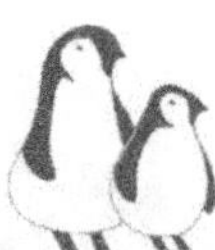

- ↑ DL_{CO}
  - Pulmonary hemorrhage
  - Polycythemia
  - L → R cardiac shunt
- DL_{CO} normal
  - ↓ lung volumes
  - Extrapulmonary disease

Abbreviations: COPD, chronic obstructive pulmonary disease; DL_{CO} diffusing capacity of lung for CO (carbon monoxide); FEV1, force expiratory volume in 1 sec; FVC, forced vital capacity

Pulse Oximetry

- Pulse oximeter % O_2 desaturation (oxyhemoglobin)
  - COPD
  - Pulmonary fibrosis
  - Exercise-associated desaturation
- Measures O_2 saturation in peripheral capillaries
- Reflects arterial O_2 saturation within < 3%

➢ Limitations

- False positive (falsely low reading)
  - Vasoconstriction
  - Hypoperfusion
- False negative (falsely higher reading)
  - CO poisoning (both hemoglobin and carboxyhemoglobin are measured)
- Normal, but not reflective of disorder
  - O_2 saturation by pulse oximetry may be normal, even though
  - There is ↓pO_2
  - Hypercapnic respiratory failure and patient hypoventilating

- Give the result of pulse oximeter in
  - Hypoperfusion
    - Falsely low
  - Poisoning (CO [carbon monoxide], cyanide)

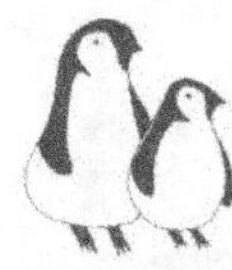

- Normal

- Methacholine (or histamine) challenge (broncho-provocation) test
  - Use when
    - History suggests asthma or exercise-induced asthma, but spirometry is normal
  - Improvement in airway obstruction
  - Asthma is excluded by normal test
  - Bronchoprovocation test
    - Normal — Rule out asthma
    - Positive — Does not prove the diagnosis of asthma

- Cardiopulmonary exercise testing exercise-induced bronchospasm

The patient with neuromuscular disease associated with weakness of the respiratory muscles has difficulty in full exhalation.

- Give the changes in PFTs (pulmonary function tests) associate with inability to achieve full exhalation.

  - ↓ TLC (total lung capacity)
  - ↑ RV (residual volume

SO YOU WANT TO BE A RESPIRATORY PHYSICIAN!

- In the context of pharyngitis in a young person, give the meaning of the Lemierre syndrome.

The **Lemierre syndrome**

- Septic thrombophlebitis of internal jugular vein
- Metastatic pulmonary infection from F. necrophorum

Spirometry

- Terms
  - FEV1 forced expiratory volume in first 1 sec on exhalation
  - FVC, forced vital capacity after deep inspiration

- Types
  - FEV1 / FVC < 70%
    - Airway obstruction
  - Spirometry with bronchodilator
    - ↑ FEV1 of ≥ 12% versus baseline, as long as
    - ↑ FEV1 > 200 mL

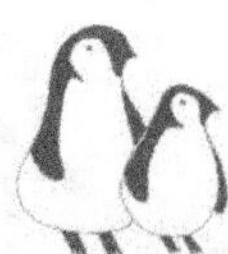

- Spirometry with flow
  - Volume loop with and without bronchodilator

	PEFR	EF shape	IF	Vol	Change AB
o Asthma	↓	Concave	↓	↓	↑
o COPD	↓	Flat	↓	↓	None
o Stenosis of trachea	↓	Flat	↓	↓	None

Abbreviations: AB, PEF after bronchodilator; IF, inspiratory flow; PEGF, peak expiratory flow rate; Vol, volume

- Note
  - Lung function
    - Best
      - Mid afternoon
    - Worse
      - Early morning

Bronchial Challenge

- Tests hyperresponsiveness to vasoconstrictor
  - Methacholine
  - Histamine
  - Monitor
- Positive test if ↓ FEV1 20% (bronchospasm) versus baseline when vasoconstrictor given

- Give the reason why mannitol is becoming the preferred agent to use in the bronchial test.

  - Asthma is a condition in which there is bronchospasm of the airways
  - Mannitol does not act directly on the airways, but instead acts as an irritant which releases endogenous mediators which are bronchoconstrictors.

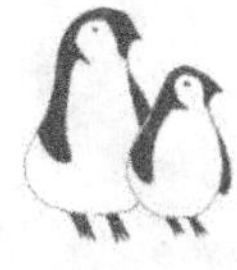

The bronchial challenge test is sensitive but not specific for the diagnosis of asthma. Thus, there are many conditions other than asthma which cause a positive test.

- Give the use of the bronchial challenge test in patient with suspected asthma.
    - Compatible symptoms, spirometry normal, negative bronchial
    - Compatible symptoms, compatible spirometry, negative bronchial challenge test
        - Test may be false negative
            - Recent use of bronchodilatory
            - Intermittent asthma (seasonal, occupational)
            - Incorrect test technique

Safety alert

Do <u>not</u> perform bronchial challenge testing in pregnancy.

Chest restriction is suspected when TLC < 80% on measurement of lung volumes.

- Give the way in which chest restriction from spirometry.
    - Chest restriction causes ↓ FEV1, ↓ FVC, but with changes in which the ratio FEV1 / FEC is either normal or increased.

Lung Volumes

- Terms

TLC, total lung capacity
IC, inspiratory capacity

ERV, expiratory reserve volume
RV, residual volume

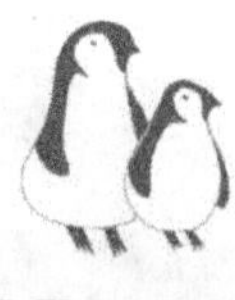

- Give the use of measuring lung volumes to distinguish between chest restriction (TLC < 80% of predicted) from parenchymal lung disease vs weakness of respiratory muscle.

Condition	TLC	RV	DLCO
o Pulmonary fibrosis (parenchymal lung disease)	↓	↓	↓
o Neuromuscular disease (weak respiratory muscle)	↓	↑	N

Diffusion Capacity

- o Diffusion capacity may be measures with small amounts of carbon monoxide (CO).
- o The diffusion capacity for CO is called DLCO.
- o The valve of DLCO depends on concentration and surface area for diffusion of CO, as well as diffusion capacity of tissue for CA, pulmonary blood pressure, and hemoglobin concentration.

Examples:

↑ DLCO

o Asthma	– Inflammation – ↑ blood volume
o Pulmonary hemorrhage	– RBC in the airspace take up ↑ CO

↓ DLCO

o Emphysema	– ↓ surface area available for gas exchange
o Fibrosis	– ↓ diffusion capacity
o Pneumonia	– Diffuse infiltration of parenchyma
o Anemia	– ↓ RBC to take up CO
o PHT (pulmonary hypertension)	– Disadvantageous diffusion gradients

Abbreviation: DLCO, diffusion capacity for carbon monoxide

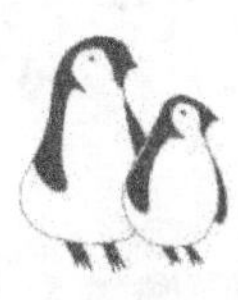

6-Minute Walk Test

- o Useful to measure O_2 saturation (by pulse oximetry) at same time as exercise
- o Follow change in distance walked in 6 min over a time interval to establish
  - Need for O_2 therapy
  - Disease progression
  - Response to therapy

Chest X-ray

- Give the systematic approach to reading a PA and lateral chest x-ray.

o General	- Date, name, age, sex - State types of studies PA and lateral - Obtain previous films for comparison - Quality of film - Rotation - Exposure - Inspiration - Any obvious abnormalities
o Bones and joints (fractures, arthritis)	- Anterior and posterior ribs - Vertebral column - Clavicles - Scapulae
o Soft tissues (calcifications, subcutaneous emphysema)	- Axillae - Breast shadows (e.g., mastectomy) - Pleura - Major and minor fissures - Costovertebral angles
o Diaphragm	- Level - Right and left hemidiaphragm - Abdominal free air
o Heart	- Size (shouldn't be > 50% the size of the cardiothoracic ratio) - Calcifications - Atrial/ventricular enlargement
o Mediastinum	- Position of trachea, aortic arch, right heart border

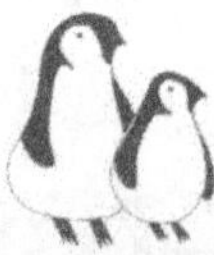

- Hila
  - Size
  - Compare right and left hilum
  - Upward/downward displacement
- Lung parenchyma
  - Nodules
  - Parenchymal density
  - Vascular abnormalities (e.g., redistribution)
- Abdomen
  - Free air
  - Gastric air bubble

Adapted form: Jugovic PJ, et al. *Saunders/ Elsevier* 2004, pages 199 to 202.

- Tricks for reading a chest X-ray

➢ Features that differentiate between the left and right hemidiaphragms in a lateral film
  - The right hemidiaphragm is usually higher than the left
  - The left hemidiaphragm is silhouetted out by the heart
  - The gastric air bubble is below the left hemidiaphragm
  - The right ribs are usually magnified since they are farther away from the film than the left ribs, so the right hemidiaphragm is the hemidiaphragm that meets the right ribs

➢ An apical lordotic view is useful when the right clavicle and first rib hinder visualization on the PA film
  - Air-space disease
    - A pathological process affecting primarily the alveoli
    - The radiological findings are Acinar shadows; air bronchograms; silhouette sign
  - Fluid (e.g., pulmonary edema); pus (e.g., pneumonia); cells (e.g., lung cancer); blood (e.g., hemorrhage); proteins (e.g., alveolar proteinosis)
  - Interstitial lung disease
    - A pathological process affecting primarily the interstitium of the lung. The radiological findings include a reticular pattern (net-like), a nodular pattern (nodules), or both
    - A differential diagnosis includes Pulmonary edema; military tuberculosis; pneumoconiosis; sarcoidosis

Adapted from: Jugovic PJ, et al. *Saunders/ Elsevier* 2004, pages 199 to 202.

- Give the meaning of Silhouette sign (actually, the "loss of silhouette").
    - The loss of normally appearing interfaces
    - Causes
        - RML consolidation – loss of right heart border
        - Lingula consolidation – loss of left heart border
        - Anterior segment of left upper lobe – loss of aortic arch

Source: Jugovic PJ, et al. *Saunders/ Elsevier* 2004, page 201.

➢ What is the typical pulmonary lobe in which disease occurs?
    - Upper – TB
    - Lower – bronchiectasis
    - Bilateral, symmetrical – pneumoconiosis

    - Lung fields – hyperlucent
    - AP chest diameter - ↑
    - Retrosternal translucent area - ↑
    - Diaphragms
        - Low
        - Flat
        - ↓ movement on ins-/ expiration
    - Pulmonary vessels – splaying (↑ angles of bifurcation)
    - Bronchi – "tram lines" because of contrast with areas of hyperinflation

Remember, the physical examination for lung collapse and fibrosis are the same. But, the chest X-ray findings are different. How?

- Give the comparison of the chest X-ray of fibrosis and collapse.

	Fibrosis	Collapse
o Distribution	Lobar or segmental	
o Homogeneous opacification	No	Yes
o Mediastinal shift	Yes	Yes
o Crowding of ribs on affected side	Yes	Yes
o Multiple cavities	Yes	Yes

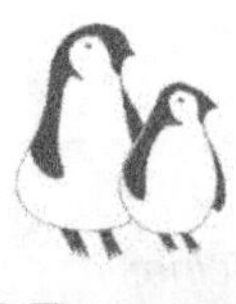

- Give the distinction between pulmonary fibrosis (PF) vs collapse (C) on a chest X-ray.

	PF	C
o Homogeneous	No	Yes
o Distribution	Lobar/ segmental	
o Shift of mediastinum	Yes	No
o Crowded ribs on affected side	Yes	No
o Multiple cavities	Yes	No

- Give the chest X-ray findings of each of the following

➢ Silicosis
  - Nodules
    - Well-defined
    - Concentric layers of fibrossi
  - Reticulation (nodules plus reticulation gives a stellate appearance)
  - Pleural fibrosis
  - Bullus/focal emphysema
  - Lymphadenopathy
  - Changes of associated – TB
  - Changes of associated – pneumoconiosis

➢ Pneumoconiosis
  - Poorly defined nodules
  - Focal emphysema
  - Upper zone nodules coalesce to form
  - Progressive massive fibrosis (PMF)
  - Cor pulmonale is commonly associated
  - Silicosis also commonly associated
  - No bullous emphysema
  - No lymph node enlargement
  - Coplan's syndrome – in men who already have or will in the future develop rheumatoid arthritis, the chest X-ray of pneumoconiosis may be atypical

➢ Asbestosis

o Lung lower lobes	- Fine moltling - Diffuse changes
o Pleura/pericardium	- Thickening (plaques) - Fuzzy outline
o Associated	- Mesothelioma - Adenocarcinoma, peripheral

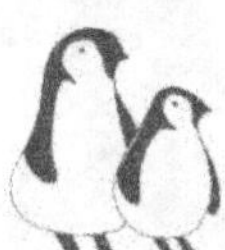

MEDIASTINAL TUMOURS

- Give causes of mediastinal tumours seen on chest X-ray.
    - Esophagus
        - Hiatus hernia
        - Corkscrew esophagus (congenital elongation)
        - Achalasia
        - Enterogenous cyst
        - Neoplasm
    - Aorta
        - Unfolding
        - Aneurysm
        - Coarctation
    - Retrosternal goiter
    - Thymoma
    - Lymphadenopathy
        - Reticulosis
        - Sarcoidosis
        - Infective (especially TB)
        - Metastasis
    - Lung cysts
        - Dermoid
        - Teratoma
        - Hydatid cysts
        - Bronchial cysts
    - Cysts
        - Pericardial cysts
        - Cardiac aneurysm or tumour
    - Miscellaneous (rare)
        - Mesothelioma
        - Lipoma
        - Sympathetic neuroma

Adapted from: Burton JL. *Churchill Livingstone* 1971, page 34.

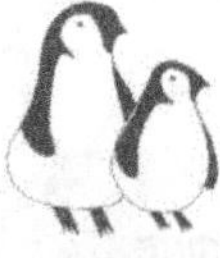

! Trick Questions !

- Give the most common causes of ring shadows (small translucent areas with white margins) seen on chest X-ray.
    - Bullae
    - Cavities
    - Cysts
    - Localized pneumothorax

- From a chest X-ray, give how can you distinguish between the homogeneous opacity caused by a collapsed basal segment of the lung, and the heart border.
    - The border of a collapsed segment may be sharp and straight
    - The heart border follows a straight line

- Under what circumstances does pleural thickening become calcified?
    - Pleural thickening becomes calcified when there is associated serous or purulent effusion.

- Under what circumstances is a hazy, homogenous opacity on chest X-ray have a well-defined border?
    - When it is due to collapse, rather than pleural thickening.

- In the context of a collapsed lung, what is Brock's syndrome?
    - Brock's syndrome is a collapsed R. middle lobe due to compression of the R. middle lobe bronchus by an enlarged lymph node.

- What is the difference between mottling and military mottling on a chest X-ray?
    - Mottling is multiple, discrete semi-confluent shadows, < 5 mm.
    - Military mottling is multiple, discrete, bilateral shadows, < 2 mm.

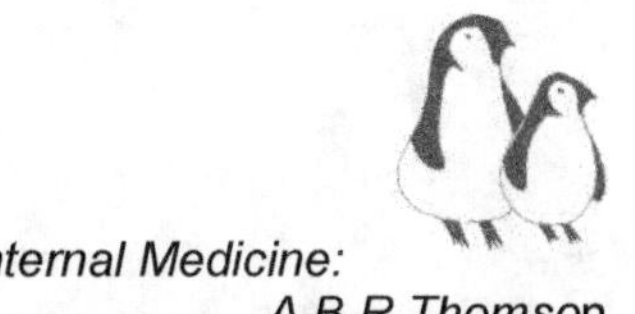

- From the site of pulmonary opacity, give the possible diagnosis for ↓ conditions.
  - Upper-lobe
    - TB (reactivation)
    - Sarcoidosis
    - Silicosis
    - Cystic fibrosis
    - Langerhans cell
    - Histiocytosis
  - Lower lobe
    - Heart failure
    - Fibrosis
    - Asbestosis
    - Pneumonia (organizing)
  - Other pulmonary testing needed for chest X-ray is of limited use in
    - PE (pulmonary embolus)
    - COPD (chronic obstructive lung disease)
    - Asthma

SO YOU WANT TO BE A PEDIATRIC RESPIROLOGIST!

- In the context of an abnormal chest X-ray in a child, what is Harrison's sulcus, and its causes.
  - Definition – Harrison sulcus is a groove which is directed downwards and outwards over the anterior chest wall
  - Causes
    - Rickets
    - Chronic chest infection

Computed Tomography (CT), **with and without Contrast**

- High resolution
- May eliminate need for lung biopsy to diagnose idiopathic pulmonary fibrosis
- CT angiography is preferred to direct pulmonary angiography or V/Q (ventilation perfusion) scan for PE (pulmonary embolus)

Positron Emission Tomography

- ↑ uptake of 18-fluorodeoxyglucose for ↑ rate of glycolysis by malignant cells
- Performance characteristics for pulmonary cancer
  - Sensitivity ~ 90%
  - Specificity ~ 85%

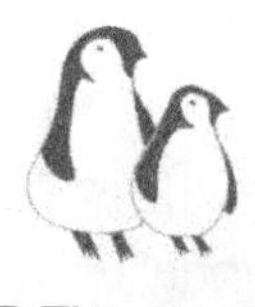

- False-positives
  - Infection e.g., TB, fungal disease
  - Inflammation e.g., Sarcoidosis
- False-negative: malignancy
  - < 1 cm diameter
  - Carcinoid
  - In situ adenocarcinoma (aka bronchioalveolar cell carcinoma)

- PET-CT highly useful to stage lung cancer, and to avoid unnecessary surgery

Bronchoscopy plus Biopsy or Lavage

- Added diagnostic yield with
  - Fluoroscopy
  - Radial ultrasound (similar staging yield as media stinoscopy)
  - EM navigation
- Lavage
  - 95% macrophages
  - Infection diagnosis, especially with immunosuppression patient
- Therapy
  - Removal of
    - Foreign body
    - Mucus
    - Tumour
  - Insertion of stent after stricture dilation

"Mediocrity is metric modulation, bringing people back (regression) to the mean."

Grandad

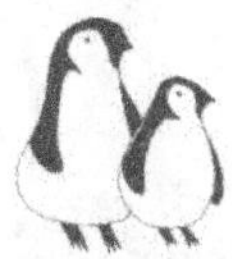

LUNG ABSCESS

➢ Clinical

- Take a focused history for the causes of lung abscess.

    - Aspiration
        - CNS
            - Coma, anesthesia, alcoholic debauch
        - Mouth
            - Oral or pharyngeal sepsis
            - Pharyngeal pouch
            - Esophageal obstruction, trachesophageal fistula
            - Drowning
            - Foreign body

    - Lung disease
        - Infection
            - TB
            - Straphylococcal
            - Friedlander infection (klebsiella)
            - Actinomycosis
            - Entameba histolytica, and other fungi
            - Secondary infection of pulmonary infarct
            - Septic emboli due to pyemia
            - Parasites, eg schistosomiasis
        - Infiltration
            - Necrotic bronchial carcinoma
            - Benign tumour
        - Ideopathic
            - Pulmonary fibrosis (interstitial lung disease)
        - Inherited/aquired cysts
        - Miscellaneous
            - Arteritis
            - Mucoviscidosis

Adapted from: Burton JL. *Churchill Livingstone* 1971, page 30.

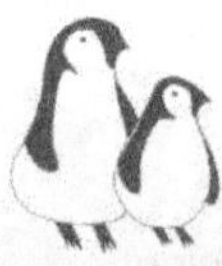

PLEURAL EFFUSION

- Causes
  - Lung
    - Infections (usually an exudates)
      - Parapneumonic (bacterial) effusions
      - Bacterial empyema
      - Tuberculosis
      - Fungi
      - Parasites
      - Viruses & mycoplasma
    - Neoplasms
      - Primary metastatic lung tumours
      - Lymphoma and leukemia
      - Benign and malignant tumours of pleura
      - Intra-abdominal tumours with ascites
    - Vascular disease
      - Pulmonary embolism
      - Wegener granulomatosis
    - Trauma
      - Hemothorax
      - Chylothorax
    - Miscellaneous
      - Drug induced effusions
  - Heart
    - Heart failure
    - Superior vena caval obstruction
    - Constrictive pericarditis
    - Post-CABG (coronary artery bypass graft)
  - GI
    - Intra abdominal diseases
      - Pancreatitis and pancreatic pseudocyst
      - Subdiaphragmatic abscess
      - Malignancy with ascites
      - Esophageal rupture
      - Intra abdominal surgery
  - Liver
    - Cirrhosis with ascites
    - Hypoalbuminemia
    - Salt retaining syndromes

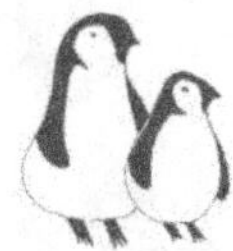

- Kidney
  - Peritoneal dialysis
  - Hydronephrosis
  - Nephrotic syndrome
  - Uremic pleuritis
- Miscellaneous
  - Meigs Syndrome
  - Myxedema
  - Familial Mediterranean fever

Adapted from: Ghosh AK. *Mayo Clinic Scientific Press* 2008, page 912.

➢ Laboratory

o Thoracentesis	- For aspiration of effusion and analysis of fluid - Only necessary when effusion is ▪ Unexplained ▪ > 1 cm (chest X-ray, fluid > 1 cm between chest wall and lung)
o Pleural fluid measurements	- Protein, or albumin concentrations - Cell counts - Biochemistry

- When the pleural effusion shows
  - LDH > 200 U/L, or > 2/3 ULN, plus
  - Pleural fluid protein/serum protein > 0.5
  - 99% accuracy for exudate (↑ vascular permeability)
  - Note: if diuretics have been used, or there are 2 processes, 1 leading to a transudate and 1 leading to an exudate, this rule of thumb may not be correct.
- Pleural fluid WBC
  - > 10,000 / mL (mostly PMNs)
    - Parapneumonic effusion, uncomplicated
    - Sudiaphragmatic abscess
    - Acute pancreatitis
  - 50,000 / mL
    - Parapneumonic effusion, completed
    - Empyema

- Criteria for transudative process causing pleural effusion
  - Usual circumstances (patient not an diuretic)
    - Total protein fluid / serum > 0.5
    - LDH (lactate dehydrogenase concentration) effusion fluid > 2/3 ULN
  - Patient on a diuretic

Characteristics of transudate $\xrightarrow{\text{diuretic}}$ Exudate

Biochemistry of pleural fluid

- Glucose
  - A low glucose concentration in pleural fluid (< 3.33 mmol/L, or 60 mg/dL) suggests TB, cancer, parapneumonic effusion, or rheumatoid disease.

- Give the prognostic significance of a low glucose concentration in pleural fluid associated with parapneumonic effusions and cancer.

  - A low pleural fluid glucose concentration suggests
    - Parapneumonic
    - Malignant effusion
      - Chest tube required
      - ↑ yield of malignant cell on cytology
      - ↑ mortality rate
      - ↓ benefit of pleurodesis
  - Triglyceride
  - Milky pleural fluid suggests chylothorax, but only about half of persons with chylothorax (pleural fluid triglyceride > 1.2 mmol/L [100 mg/dL] will have this appearance
  - The modified **Light criteria** are usually ~ 100% sensitive and 83% specific for an exudate process causing the pleural effusion: except when there is concurrent therapy with diuretics.
    - Albumin gradient between serum to pleural fluid > 1.2 g/dL, or
    - Total protein gradient between serum to pleural fluid > 3.1 g/dL (31 g/L)
    - The pathophysiological process can be transudative or exudative
    - Said another way, finding a pleural effusion in patient with HF on diuretic cannot with certainty be considered to be non-exudative
    - The exception is when the HF patient is on diuretics

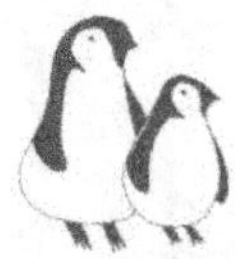

Clinical Gem

- In the patient with a pleural effusion who has been placed on a diuretic before a thoracentosis and analysis of the pleural fluid has been performed, give the way in which a trasnsudate may be differentiated from an exudate.
    - In the patient on a diuretic, a transudate is suggested by
        - Total protein gradient (serum-pleural fluid total protein) > 31 g/L (3.1 g/dL), or
        - Total albumin gradient (serum-pleural fluid albumin concentration) > 12 g/L (1.2 g/dL)

- Give the characteristics of pleural fluid which suggest empyema.
    - pH < 7.20
    - Glucose effusion/blood < 50%
    - LDH > 1000 U/L
    - ↑ WBC > 50,000 / mL
    - Gram stain/culture positive

When patient with a transxudate is given a diuretic, the charateristics of the pleural fluid look more like that of an exudate, i.e.,

- Total protein pleural fluid/serum < 0.5
- LDH pleural fluid < 2/3 ULN

➢ Cell counts in pleural fluid

- RBC
    - Hemothorax
        - Suspect hematocrit > 50% in pleural fluid
- WBC
    - > 10 x 10^9 / L (> 10,000 WBC per mL)
    - Lymphocyte predominant
        - TB
        - Cancer
        - Transudate (WBC transudates are normally predominant in lymphocytes)
    - Eosinophils
        - Air
        - Blood
        - Infection, inflammation, medications
        - Idiopathic (~ 1/3)

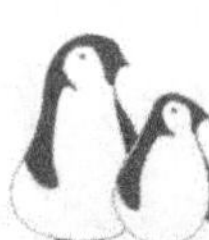

TB-Associated Pleural Effusion

- Give the approximate percentages of patients diagnosed to have TB of the lung in the patient with a pleural effusion.

Test	% of patients
o Positive PPD (purified protein derivative) test, plus lymphocyte predominant exudate	
– TB until proven otherwise	
o Biopsy of pleura	
– Granulomas	80-90%
– Positive culture	25%
o Pleural fluid	
– Positive smear	< 5%
– Adenosine deaminase < 40 U/L	~ 0%*

*adenosine deaminase < 40 U/L has a negative predictive value of ~ 100%

- Give the measuring adenosine deaminase (AD) in patient with pleural effusion which is suspected to be TB.

o AD > 70 U/L	o TB is likey
o AD < 40 U/L	o TB is unlikely

Malignancy-Associated Pleural Effusions

- Give the approximate percentages (%) of patients diagnosed as having a malignancy-associated pleural effusion, depending upon the number (#) of taps.
  - o Thoracentesis
    - \# 1 65%
    - \# 2 92%
    - \# 3 97%
  - o Pleural biopsy thorascopic 90% sensitive

- Give treatment options for the **treatment** of malignant pleural effusion.
  - o Repeated therapeutic thoracentesis
  - o Chemical pleurodesis
  - o Indwelling pleural catheter, tunneled

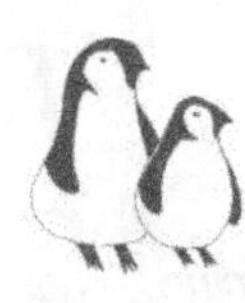

LUNG INFECTION

Pneumonia

➢ Clinical

- Give the performance characteristics of physical examination for pneumonia.

The PLRs for crackles and wheezes for the diagnosis of pneumonia are each < 2.0

Finding	PLR
o General appearance	
- Cachexia	4.0
o Vital signs	
- Temperature > 37.8°C	2.0
- Respiratory rate > 28/min	2.0
o Lung findings	
- Percussion dullness	3.0
- Diminished breath sounds	2.3
- Bronchial breath sounds	3.3
- Egophony	4.1

Abbreviation: PLR, positive likelihood ratio

Adapted from: McGee SR. *Saunders/Elsevier* 2007, Box 29.1, page 352.

CLINICAL TIPS

- At an early stage of pneumonia, before consolidation occurs there may be
  - Mottling
  - Homogeneous opacity
- Homogeneous opacity may be caused by
  - Homogeneous opacity
  - Collapse
  - Effusion
- Deviation of heart or trachea excludes uncomplicated pneumonia
- Bronchopneumonia is usually bilateral

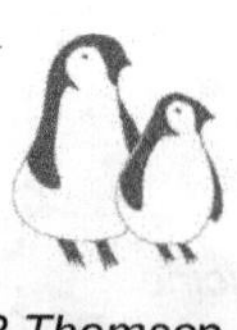

➢ Diagnosis

Useful background: Multivariate findings for adult pneumonia

Add points for the presence of findings as follows:
Rhinorrhea= 2 points; sore throat= -1; night sweats = 1; myalgias = 1; sputum all day= 1; respiratory rate > 25/min=2; temperature $\geq$37.8°C (100°F) = 2

Threshold score	LR
$\geq$3	14
$\geq$1	5.0
$\geq$ -1	1.5
< -1	0.22

Score= -3.095 + 1.214 (cough) + 1.007 x (fever) + 0.823 x (crackles)
Each variable is coded as 1 if present, 0 if absent
Probability of pneumonia = 1/(1 + e score)

Source: Simel DL, et al. *JAMA* 2009, Table 40-5, page 536.

"A pessimist sees the difficulty in every opportunity;
An optimist sees the opportunity in every difficulty."
Sir Winston Churchill

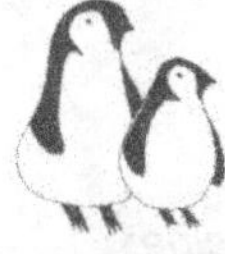

COMMUNITY-ACQUIRED PNEUMONIA (CAP)

- Definition
  - "………an acute pneumonia occurring in persons who have not been hospitalized recently and are not living in facilities such as nursing homes"
  - A wide spectrum of severity, and the risks of morbidity and mortality may be estimated and stratified based on the need for hospitalization, IRVS (intensive respiratory or vasomotor support) or risk of death:
  - PSI (pneumonia-specific severity of illness) score
    - Predicts need for hospital admission
  - SMRT-CO
    - Predicts risk of death
  - CURB-65
    - Predicts risk of death

Note: with CAP patients who require hospitalization, the MR (mortality rate) is 10%; for those requiring admission to ICU, the MR is 40%

Useful background: Poor prognostic factors in patients with community-acquired pneumonia (CAP)

- Demography
  - Age over 65 years
- Coexisting conditions such as
  - Cardiac failure
  - Renal failure
  - Chronic obstructive pulmonary disease (COPD)
  - Malignancy
- Clinical
  - Respiratory rate > 30 per min
  - Hypotension (systolic blood pressure < 90 mmHg or diastolic pressure < 60 mmHg)
  - Temperature > 38.3°C
  - Impaired mental status (stupor, lethargy, disorientation or coma)
  - Extrapulmonary infection (e.g., septic arthritis, meningitis)

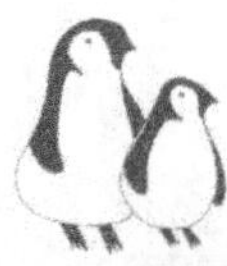

- Prognosis
  - MR (mortality rate)
    - Outpatient 5%
    - Inpatient 10%
    - ICU patients 30%

- Give the predictors of hospital mortality of pneumonia

Finding		PLR
o General appearance	- Abnormal mental status	2.8
o Vital signs	- Respiratory rate > 30/min	2.1
	- Systolic blood pressure < 90 mmHg	10.0
	- Heart rate > 100/min	2.1
	- Hyporthermia	3.5

Abbreviation: PLR, positive likelihood ratio

Adapted from: McGee SR. *Saunders/Elsevier* 2007, Box 29.2, page 355.

- Probability of pneumonia from clinical finding increases
- Count the number of findings present
  - Absence of asthma
  - Temperature $\geq$37.8°C (100°F)
  - Heart rate > 100/min
  - ↓ breath sounds
  - Crackles

Number of Findings	Probability, % (baseline prevalence 5%)
5	50
4	25
3	20
2	3
1	1
0	<1

Source: Simel DL, et al. *JAMA* 2009, Table 40-6, page 536.

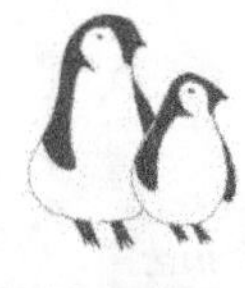

- Perform a focused physical examination for complications of pneumonia.
    - Skin
        - Rash
        - Erthema multiform (EM)
        - Steven-Johnson syndrome-(S-JS)
    - Lung
        - Abscess
        - Empyema
        - ARDS
    - Heart
        - Pericarditis
        - Myocarditis
    - Blood
        - Septicemia
        - Hemolysis – hemolytic syndrome
        - DIC – autoimmune*
    - Kidney
        - Glomerulonephritis*
        - Renal failure
    - Liver
        - Hepatitis*
    - MSK
        - Arthralgia/arthritis*
        - Myositis
        - Rhabdomyolysis
    - CNS, PNS
        - Confusion
        - Coma
        - Encephalitis
        - Aseptic meningitis
        - Transverse myelitis
        - GBS (Guillain-Barre syndrome)

Abbreviations: ARDS, adult respiratory distress syndrome; CNS, central nervous system; DIC, disseminated intravascular coagulation; EM, erythema multiforme; PNS, peripheral nervous system; S-JS, Stevens- Johnson syndrome

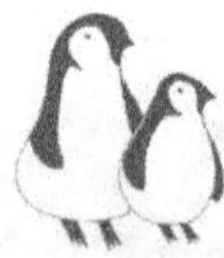

- **Community-Acquired Pneumonia (CAP)**

➢ Risks

- Give 6 factors which provide ↑ risk for CAP.
  - Predisposition
    - Lifestyle
      - Smoking
      - Alcohol
    - Malnutrition
    - Lung
      - Chronic bronchitis
      - COPD
      - Bronchitis
      - Cystic fibrosis
    - CV system
      - CV disease
    - Liver disease
      - Cirrhosis
    - Long-term use of corticosteroids

➢ Investigations
- Hematocrit < 30%
- White cell count < 4000 or > 30 000 per mm^3
- Azotemia
- Arterial blood gas < 60 mmHg while breathing room air
- Chest radiograph showing multiple lobe involvement
- Rapid spread or pleural effusion

➢ Common microbial pathogens: *Staph. Aureus, Legionella, Strep. Pneumonaie*

Adapted from: Baliga RR. *Saunders/Elsevier* 2007, pages 273 and 281; McGee SR. *Saunders/Elsevier* 2007, Box 27-2.

- Bacteriology
  - Overall commonest
    - Streptococcus pneumonia
    - Haemophilus influenza
    - Moraxella catarrhalis
  - Chronic medical disease gram-negative
  - Chronic liver disease
  - Alcoholism

  } Enteric bacilli

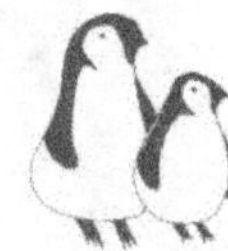

- Klebsiella pneumonia
- Outpatients
  - Mycoplasm pneumonia
  - Chlamydophilia
- Structural lung disease
  - Pseudomonas aeruginosa
- Summer time
- Travellers

} Legionella

Following influenza
Cavity pneumonia
CA-MRSA)
SSTI (CA-MRSAIVDU)

} S. aureus, including (community-associated methicillin-resistant S. aureus)

- Virology
  - Influenza
  - Parainfluenza
  - RSV (respiratory syncytial virus)
  - Adenovirus (especially type 14)

Abbreviations: COPD, chronic obstructive pulmonary disease; SSTI, skin and soft tissue infection; IVDU, intravenous drug user

- Give the bacterial cause of CAP (community-acquired pneumonia) which

Question	Choice of Pathogen
o Does not require contact with an infected person	- Legionella pneunophilia
o Does not occur in persons who wear dentures	- Anaerobes
o Common in persons	
- With bronchiectasis	- Pseudomonas aeruginosa
- Who work on an animal farm	- Coxiella burnetii
- Who keep a bat as a pet	- Histoplasma

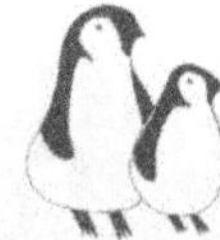

Question	Choice of Pathogen
o Occur in	
- SW USA	- Coccidioides
- SE Asia	- Burkholderia pseudomallei

Abbreviations: SE, South East; SW, South West

- Give the criteria to determine hospital admission in the patient with pneumonia.

  - o Any of the below should result in admission:
    - Respiratory rate >28/min
    - Systolic BP <90 mmHg or 30 mmHg below baseline
    - Delirium
    - Hypoxia: Oxygen sat <90% or pO2 of <60 mmHg on room air
    - Unstable co-morbid illness e.g.,: renal failure, CHF
    - Lobar multi pneumonia
    - Pleural effusion >1cm, and has features of a complicated parapneumonic effusion

- Give the typical signs of pulmonary infarction seen on chest X-ray.

  - o Opacity
    - ▪ Round, triangular or linear
    - ▪ Maybe absent, especially with middle lobe collapse
    - ▪ May be absent for the first 24 hours after onset of pleuritic chest pain
  - o Pleural effusion
  - o Elevation of hemidiaphragm

➢ Investigation

- o Hospitalized but not in the ICU, diagnostic testing is recommended for
  - Lung
    - ▪ Failure of outpatient antibiotics
    - ▪ Cavity infiltrates
    - ▪ COPD
    - ▪ Bronchitis
    - ▪ CF (cystic fibrosis)
  - Liver
    - ▪ Alcoholism
    - ▪ Cirrhosis

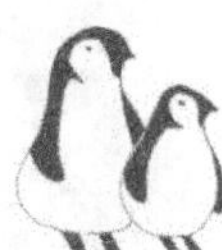

- Hematology
  - Leucopenia
  - Asplenia (structural or functional)
- Blood cultures (positive ~ 10%)
- Sputum/endotracheal aspirate
- Thoracentesis for effusion
  - Upright CHX (chest X-ray) effusion filling ≥ hemithorax
  - Lateral decubitus CHX, effusion > 1 cm
- Urine antigen testing

Organism	Sensitivity	Specificity
Pneumococcal	70%	96%
Legionella (L. pneumophilia, serogroup 1)	70% to 90%	99%

➢ Risk assessment

- Give a definition of severe CAP (community-acquired pneumonia), and state the necessary infection-related (microbiological) investigations.
  - Definition severe CAP: "….. CAP in a patient necessitating admission to an intensive care unit or transfer to an intensive care unit 24 hours of admission" (MKSAP 16, Infectious disease 2012, page 174)
  - Suggested investigations (microbiological)

- Sputum from endotracheal aspirate	▪ Gram stain ▪ Culture
- Blood	▪ Culture
- Urine	▪ Antigen assays for – Legionella – Streptococcus pneumoniae

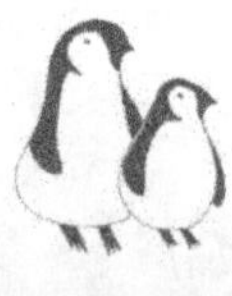

The severity of CAP is assessed using the **CURB-65 criteria**. We all use CURB-65 all the time, but do you know what it stands for?

- Give the CURB-65 criteria.
  - ≥ 65 yr
  - ↑ respiratory rate
  - ↓ blood pressure
  - Confusion
  - Uremia

IDSA / ATS Minor Criteria for Severe Community-Acquired Pneumonia

- Clinical Criteria
  - Confusion (new-onset disorientation to person, place, or time)
  - Hypothermia (core temperature < 36 °C [96.8 °F])
  - Respiration rate ≥ 3 0/min
  - Hypotension necessitating aggressive fluid resuscitation
  - Multi-lobar pulmonary infiltrates

- Laboratory Criteria
  - Arterial PO_2 / Fio_2 ratio ≤ 250
  - Leukopenia (< 4000 cells / µL [4.0 x 10^9 / L])
  - Thrombocytopenia (< 100,000 / µL [10 x 10^9 / L])
  - Blood urea nitrogen > 20 mg/dL (7.1 mmol/L)

- The British Thoracic Society severity score is based on four criteria.
  CURB
  - **C**onfusion
  - **U**rea > 7mmol/L
  - **R**espiratory rate > 30/min* (without underlying lung disease)
  - **B**lood pressure <60 mmHg diastolic or systolic <90 mmHg

Mortality with no features is 2.4%, with one feature 8%, with two 23%, with three 33% and all four features, 83%.

Source: McGee SR. *Saunders/Elsevier* 2007, page 354.

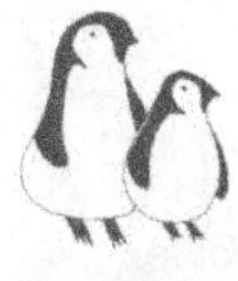

- Treatment
  - Site of care
    - Determination if hospitalization is indicated based on scoring of patients' severity (which reflects patient mortality rate)
      - CURB-65 score (1 point for each)
        - ≥ 65 yrs
        - Confusion
        - RR ≥ 30 / min
        - SBP < 90 mm Hg
        - DBP < 70 mm Hg

Score	Site of care
0-1	Outpatient
≥ 2	Hospital
≥ 3	ICU

Abbreviations: DBP, diastolic blood pressure; RR, respiratory rate; SBP, systolic blood pressure

      - PSI (pneumonia severity index) decision support tool http://pda.ahrq.gov/clinic/psi/psicalc.asp
      - Note:
        - Psychosocial factors will also play a part regarding determining role of hospitalization
        - In patients who are initially admitted to hospital (URB ≥ 2) and who deteriorate and are then transferred to ICU (CURB ≥ 3), the mortality rate is > 50%
        - In addition to CURB score ≥ 3, the decision to be admitted to hospital can be estimated the IDSA / ATS guidelines
  - Antibiotics

- Give the reason why guideline-concordant empiric antibiotics rather than pathogen-directed therapy are recommended for treatment of CAP (for outpatients, but not ICU patients).
  - There is no demonstrable difference in outcome (let us say again, except for CAP patients in the ICU).
    - Empiric antibiotic therapy should be started within 4 hrs of presentation
    - Choice of antibiotics depends upon the site of care (please see above), and the likelihood of the underlying pathogens
    - Outpatients, otherwise healthy
      - Azithromycin, clarithromycin, or erythromycin, or
      - Doxycycline

Adapted from:MKSAP 16, Infectious disease 2012, Table 14, page 21.

- For the patient with CAP who is well enough to be treated as an outpatient, given 5 conditions which ↑ risk of drug-resistant S. pneumonia and therefore influence the choice of empiric antibiotics to be used.
  - > 65 yrs
  - B-lactam antibiotics used within past 6 mon
  - Alcoholism
  - Immunosuppression
  - Comorbidities (e.g., diabetes)
  - Recent exposure to a child in daycare
  - Risk factors for drug-resistant S. pneumonia
    - Moxifloxacin, gemifloxacin, levofloxacin (macrolide)
    - Amoxicillin-clavulanate, cefpodoxime, cefuroxime, plus
    - Macrolide (see above), or
    - Doxycycline
  - In patients (ward, or ICU, depending upon CURB score and IDSA / ATS criteria; and as well influenced by confined microbial cause)
    - Initially, antibiotics are given IV until patient is stable
    - Selection of empiric antibiotics for CAP patient admitted to hospital depend upon their risk or sputum demonstrated
      - P. aerugenosa
      - CA-MRSA
  - Ceftriaxone or cefotaxime plus azithromycin or doxycycline
  - If this CAP were to occur after an influenza-like illness, then CAP due to MRSA (methicillin-resistant Staphylococcus) would be suspected, and to the above regimen would be added vancomycin.
  - What is the typical history of the patient who develops bacterial pneumonia after a viral infection is an initial viral syndrome which improves, then suddenly worsens?
- For guidance for the selection of antibiotic therapy for CAP in inpatients, please see a standard medical textbook, or a recent review such as UptoDate or MKSAP 16, Infectious disease 2012, Table 16, page 22.
- For guidance for the selection of pathogen-specific antibiotic therapy for CAP, please see standard medical textbook, or a recent review such as UptoDate or MKSAP 16, Infectious disease 2012, Table 17, page 23.
- For bacteremia pneumococcal pneumonia, combined β-Lactam and macrolide therapy is beneficial.

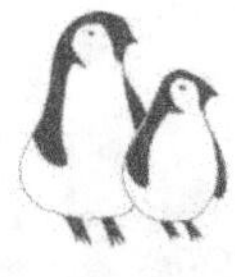

- Route of antibiotics
  - A Reminder: the patient is initially given antibiotics IV (intravenous) until the patient is stable (i.e., fit to be set home from hospital)
  - Once stable, the patient is switched to oral therapy of the treated CAP patient

- Give the criteria for stability which would allow for them to be switched from IV to po therapy, and to be discharged home (unless there are other medical issues besides the CAP, or compounding psychosocial issue).
  - Temperature ≤ 37.8 °C (100 °F)
  - RR ≤ 24 / min
  - PR ≤ 24 / min
  - SBP ≥ 90 mm Hg
  - % O_2 sat ≥ 90%, or
  - pO_2 ≥ 60 mmHg

Note:
  - CAP patient with bacteremia may take longer to become stable
  - If time to stability > 3 days, there is ↑ rate of
    - Rehospitalisation
    - Death

Abbreviations: PR, pulse rate; RR, respiratory rate; SAT, saturation; SBP, systolic blood pressure

- Duration of antibiotics
  - Usually, 7 days in total
  - Spread circumstances for longer therapy
  - Prolonged interval to be "stable", as defined above
  - Cavity pneumonia
  - Infection with
    - S. aureus
    - P. aeruginosa

- Vaccination program
  - Pneumococcus
  - Influenza

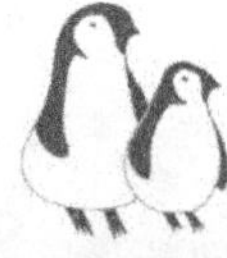

- Follow-up
  - Outpatient visit within 14 days of hospitalization, or earlier if time for patient to become stable was > 3 days
    - 1/3 of patients may continue to have symptoms for a month
    - Continue to follow as per usual guidelines patients with CAP-associated guidelines such as COPD, bronchiectasis, or CV disease
  - Chest X-ray within 8 weeks of treatment
    - Smokers
    - > 40 yrs
    - Note: ~ 10% of persons with CAP who are hospitalized have underlying lung cancer

- Give the management of a parapneumonic effusion which develops a pleural effusion.

  - Small
    - If patient
      - Responding to cefotaxime plus azithromycin, continue
      - Not responding, switch to
        - Cefepime plus vancomycin

  - Large
    - Definition
      - ≥ half of hemithorax filled with fluid on upright view of chest X-ray
      - > 1 cm of fluid on lateral decubitus view of chest X-ray
    - Treatment
      - Thoracentesis plus antibiotics

- Give the empiric therapy for Pseudomanas aeruginosa pneumonia.

  - Anti-pseudomonal β-lactam agent with pneumococcal coverage cefepime, imipenem, meropenem, or
  - Piperacillin-tazobactam plus ciprofloxacin or levofloxacin, or
  - An anti-pseudominal β-lactam with pneumococcal coverage plus an aminoglycoside plus a respiratory fluoroquinolone
  - For persons with severe β-lactam allergy aztreonam

VAP (ventilator-associated pneumonia) is associated with the risk of pneumonia in patients who are already severely ill. Reducing this risk is not associated with antibiotic prophylaxis or early tracheostomy.

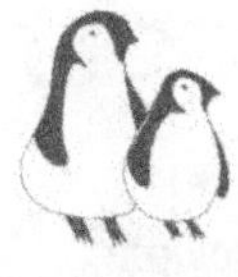

- Give the current standard of care to ↓ risk of developing VAP.
    - Elevate to head of the bed by 30°
    - Chlorhexidine mouth washes
    - Early weaning off ventilator (daily assessments to determine if the patient is ready to be weaned from the ventilator)

- Give the one antibiotic which is sensitive against both MRSA pneumonia, VAP (ventilator-associated pneumonia), VRE (vancomycin-resistant enterococci).
    - For MRSA, VRE and VAP, linezolid is recommended

SO YOU WANT TO BE A PULMONARY PHYSICIAN!

- In the context of the patient with pneumonia complicated by a cavity, give the likely causative organism based on the appearance of the cavity.

Air-fluid level	– Staphylococci – Anaerobes – Gram-negative bacilli
No air-fluid level	– Tuberculosis – Fungal infection

- **Hospital-Acquired Pneumonia** (HAP) **and Ventilator-Associated Pneumonia** (VAP)

➢ Definitions
- HAP
    - Symptoms of pneumonia plus new / progressive infiltration on chest X-ray ≥ 48 hr after hospitalization
- VAP
    - A subset of HAP, occurring > 48 after endotracheal intubation
    - Pneumonia beginning ≥ 48 hr after endothelial intubation

➢ Diagnosis
- Aspirate lower respiratory treat after mini-bronchoalveolar lavage (BAL), plus brushing using protected specimen brush

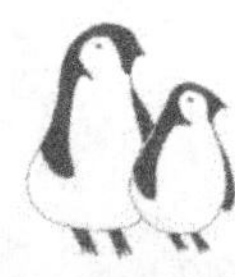

- Thresholds for diagnosing VAP
  - BAL > 10^4 CFU/mL sample
  - Brushing > 10^3 CFU/mL sample

- Treatment
  - Depends upon risk for MDRO (multi-drug-resistant organisms)
  - Risk factors for MDRO
    - Hospitalization
      - ≥ 5 days
      - From a healthcare facility
    - Drugs (recent)
      - Antibiotics
      - Immunosuppressants
  - No MDRO risks
    - Ceftriaxone, or
    - Levofloxacin
  - MDRO risk
    - Vancomycin, plus
    - Cefepime or ceftriaxone

- Give the rational for the antibiotic selection for HAP/VAP associated with risk of MDRO.
  - Vancomycin – MRSA
  - Cefepime or ceftriaxone – Pseudomonas aeruginosa

Useful background: Pneumonia-specific Severity of Illness (PSI) Score

Patient characteristic	Points assigned
- Males	Age (years)
- Females	Age (years) minus 10
- Nursing home resident	10
Comorbid illness	
- Neoplastic disease	30
- Liver disease	20
- Heart failure	10
- Cerebrovascular disease	10
- Renal disease	10

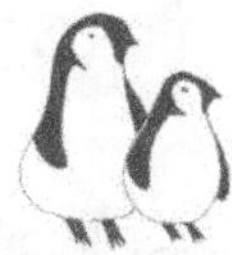

- Physical examination findings

– Altered mental status	20
– Respiratory rate ≥30 breaths/min	20
– Systolic blood pressure <90 mm Hg	20
– Temperature <35°C or ≥40°C	15
– Pulse ≥125 beats/min	10

- Laboratory findings

– Arterial pH <7.35	30
– Blood urea nitrogen >11 mmol/L	20
– Sodium <130 mmol/L	20
– Glucose ≥14 mmol/L	10
– Hematocrit <30%	10
– Partial pressure of arterial oxygen <60 mm Hg	10
– Pleural effusion	10

Reproduced with permission: Therapeutics Choices. Sixth Edition. Ottawa, Canada: *Canadian Pharmacist Association* 2012, page 1396.

➢ Complications

- Give complications of pneumonia.

  - General
    - Septicemia
    - Multi-organ failure
    - Hemolytic syndrome
    - Death
  - CNS – central and peripheral nervous systems
  - Heart – pericarditis, myocarditis
  - Lung abscess
    - Empyema
    - Adult respiratory distress syndrome
  - Atypical pneumonia
    - Typical pneumonia is caused by pneumococcus (*S. pneumonia)*
    - Atypical pneumonia is caused by *Mycoplasma, Legionella. Chlamydia, Coxiella*, etc.
    - The clinical picture in atypical pneumonia is dominated by constitutional symptoms, such as fever and headache, rather than by respiratory symptoms

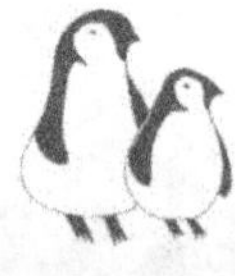

- Kidney
  - Renal failure
  - Glomerulonephritis
- Liver – hepatitis
- Blood
  - Disseminated intravascular coagulation (DIC)
  - Autoimmune hemolytic anemia
- MSK
  - Arthralgia and arthritis
- Skin
  - Non-specific rash
  - Erythema multiforme
  - Stevens-Johnson syndrome

Adapted from: Baliga RR. *Saunders/Elsevier* 2007, page 272.

- Give causes of slow resolution or recurrence of pneumonia.
  - Bronchial obstruction
    - Neoplasm
    - Aspiration of foreign body
    - Compression of bronchus
    - Bronchiectasis (of the infected lobe)
    - Pulmonary embolism with infarctions
  - General
    - Antibiotic
    - Decreased host resistance
    - Cachexia
    - Agranulocytosis
    - Immunoglobulin defects etc.
  - Lung
    - Formation of abscess, empyema or serous effusion
    - Other causes of pulmonary fibrosis
  - Pharynx/hypopharynx
    - Pharyngeal pouch with 'spilling'
    - Zenker diverticulum
  - Metabolic
    - Diabetes
  - Immune deficiency

Adapted from: Burton JL. *Churchill Livingstone* 1971, page 28; Baliga RR. *Saunders/Elsevier* 2007, page 272.

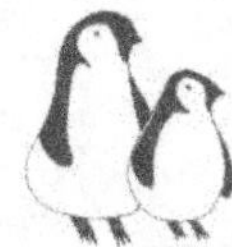

! Trick Question !

Why may the middle lobe collapse and disappear in some persons suffering from a pulmonary infarction?

- o The right middle bronchus may collapse, the middle lobe then collapses, and retracts towards the hilum
- o The remaining normal lung lobes dilate (compensatory emphysema), and obscure the collapsed middle lobe.

SO YOU WANT TO BE A RESPIROLOGIST!

- In the setting of the patient with a lung collapse, give the meaning of the Brock syndrome.
- o The Brock syndrome is lung collapse due to compression of the right middle lobe bronchus by an enlarged lymph node, often from TB.

Source: Baliga RR. *Saunders/Elsevier* 2007, page 292.

INFLUENZA VIRUS A, B

➢ Demography

- Give the groups of persons who are at high risk of developing severe disease from influenza virus, and must be considered for vaccination or treatment if not vaccinated.
  - o Age > 64 yr
  - o Pregnant or within 2 wk of delivery
  - o First Nations persons
  - o Chronic disease e.g., diabetes; lung heart, kidney, blood disorders
  - o Immunosuppressed

➢ Prophylaxis

- o Immunization
- o Antivirals
  - o Zanamivir
  - o Oseltamivir

  } for 2 wk after immunization in staff members of an institution with an epidemic

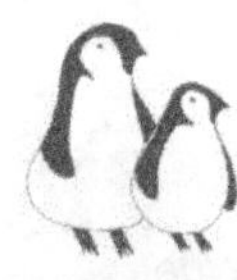

- Treatment
  - Zanamivir
  - Oseltamivir

  } hospitalized patients with ↑ risk for severe disease

Therapeutic Alerts

Zanamir is effective to be used for **influenza** A or B viral infection.

- Give the major complication of this antiviral agent.
  - Because this drug may cause severe bronchospasm, it is **not** given (contraindicated) in persons with heart or lung disease.

It is well recognized that the vaccine for influenza is live attenuated virus, and must not be given to some groups of persons, to whom the influenza vaccine must not be given.

- Give another major group of persons to whom the influenza vaccine must not be given.
  - Household and other close contacts of immunosuppressed persons must not receive the live attenuated influenza A/B vaccine

---

- Prophylaxis

- Give the recommended persons to receive seasonal influenza immunization.
  - Persons at high risk for influenza-related complications
    - Adults and children ≥6 month of age with chronic cardiac or respiratory disorders (includes asthma, bronchopulmonary dysplasia, cystic fibrosis and COPD) requiring regular medical follow-up
    - All residents of nursing homes and other long-term care facilities
    - All persons ≥65 y of age
    - Adults and children ≥6 month of age with any of the following chronic disorders:
      - Diabetes mellitus or other metabolic disorder
      - Cancer
      - Immunosuppression (due to underlying disease or treatment)

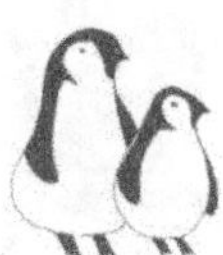

	▪ Renal disease ▪ Anemia ▪ Hemoglobinopathies – Children and adolescents (6 month-18 year of age) requiring chronic ASA therapy – Pregnant women (all trimesters) – HealthY children 6-23 months
○ Persons capable of transmitting influenza to those at high risk of influenza-related complications	– Healthcare workers and other personnel (e.g., volunteers, housekeeping staff) who have significant contact with those in the above-mentioned high-risk groups, regardless of the practice setting – Adults and children ≥6 months of age who are household contacts of those at high risk of influenza-related complications. – This includes household contacts of children <6 month old who are at high risk of complications from influenza but for whom there is no currently licensed vaccine. Pregnant women should be immunized if they are expected to deliver during influenza season; they will become household contacts of their newborn. – Those providing regular childcare to children age 0-23 month, whether in or out of the home
○ Other	– People who provide essential community services, e.g., police officers and fire fighters – People who are in direct contact with avian influenza-infected poultry during culling operations
○ Additional considerations in 2010-2011	– Persons who are morbidly obese (BMI ≥40) – First Nations persons – Healthy children age 2-4 y

Reproduced with permission: Therapeutics Choices. Sixth Edition. Ottawa, Canada: Canadian Pharmacist Association 2012, Table 1, page 1382.

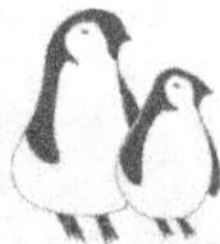

- In the context of infections with influenza virus, give the difference between antigenic drifts and antigenic shifts.

Terminology	Antigenic changes	Outbreaks
o Antigenic drift	- Minor gene mutations and recombinations	▪ Local
o Antigenic shift	- Major changes in surface glycoproteins	▪ Pandemic

➢ Treatment
- o Antibiotics for secondary bacterial pneumonia
- o Neurominidase inhibitors
  - Zanamivir
  - Oseltamivir
- o Vaccination annually (Pneumococcal)

"The decisions of our present are the architects of our present."

Dan Brown

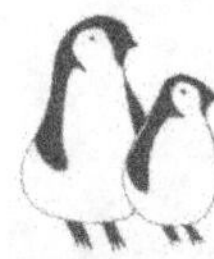

MYCOBACTERIUM TUBERCULOSIS

- Primary infection
  - Inhalation of respiratory droplets takes the Mycobacterium tuberculosis acid-fast bacillus to the terminal airways where macrophages ingest the mycobacterium which multiplies and may spread through blood or lymphatics to other tissues

- Latent TB Infection (LTBI)
  - Develops from primary infection
  - Asymptomatic, non-contagious disease
  - Suggested by
    - Positive Mantoux tuberculin skin test / TST
      - Delayed type hypersensitivity response to purified protein derivative
    - Positive interferon-γ release assays (IGRAs)

- Primary progressive TB
  - Progression: primary → LTBI → primary progressive (in 10% overall when untreated)
  - Risk factors for progression of either primary infection or LTBI progressive TBI immune suppression
    - HIV
    - Corticosteroids
    - Anti-TNF drugs
    - Malnutrition
    - Chronic kidney disease
    - Diabetes
    - Cancer

- Diagnosis
  - TST (tuberculin skin test)
  - Smear/histology
    - Acid fast bacilli identified
  - Special studies
    - IGRA (interferon γ release assay)
    - NAA (nucleic acid amplification)
    - Pleural fluid adenosine deaminase

Adapted from: MKSAP 16, Infectious disease 2012, Table 22, page 33.

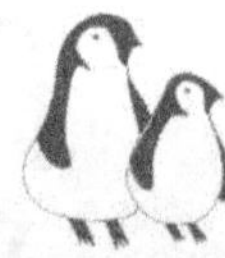

Tubercuin Skin Test (aka Mantoux Skin Test)

Note: for persons having annual serial TST, if the inclination ↑ ≥ 10 mm over 2 yr, then the test is positive.

- Give 6 causes for false-negative and/or –positive TST.

  - False-negative TST
    - Active TB (20% of active TB patients have negative TST)
    - < 6 yr old
    - Recent TB infection
    - Overwhelming
    - TB infection
    - Recent viral infection
    - Recent vaccination with live virus
    - Anergy

  - False-positive TST
    - BCG vaccination
    - Non-TB mycobacterial infection

- Give 10 high risk categories of persons who require a chest x-ray when their TST (tuberculin skin test) is ≥ 10 mm.

  - Demography
    - Children < 4 yr
    - Newborns to adolescents exposed to high-risk adults
    - Immigration < 5 yr from high risk country

  - Setting
    - IVDU (IV drug users)
    - High risk living/working conditions
  - Comorbidities
    - Diabetes
    - Chronic renal disease
    - Silicosis
    - Cancer
      - Head and neck
      - Lung
      - Lymphoproliferative disorders
    - Weight loss and
      - Gastrectomy
      - Jejunioleal bypass

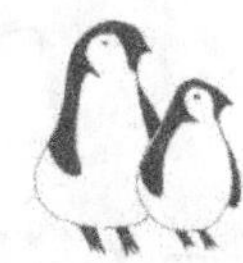

SO YOU WANT TO BE AN ID SPECIALIST!

- In the context of using the Mantoux tuberculin skin test (TST) to diagnose LTBI or active TB infection, give the meaning of "booster effect", and give 3 associated conditions.
    - The booster effect is a TST which becomes positive several weeks rather than 2-3 days after injection of the PPD (purified protein derivative).
    - Causes of booster effect include
        - Old age
        - Remote exposure to TB
        - Previous BCG vaccination
        - Non-tuberculosis mycobacterial infection

Abbreviations: CSF, cerebrospinal fluid; UTI, urinary tract infection

Test Yourself

A middle-aged non-smoking woman with no previous lung disease presents with pulmonary but no systemic symptoms, and CT chest demonstrates multiple discrete nodules in the middle lobe and lingular areas. One sputum culture is positive and one is negative for MAC (mycobacterium avium complex).

- Give the next management action.
    - NTM (non-tuberculous mycobacteria) such as MAC may occur in sputum and one sputum culture positive for MAC does not prove that the infection is active and represents the explanation for the person's symptoms.
    - If a second culture were positive, then the predictive value is adequate to initiate treatment. However, in this patient, there are both positive and negative cultures.
    - The index of suspicion is help for MAC (middle-aged women, discrete nodules on chest CT, involvement of middle lobe and lingual area), that the next step would be
        - Culture bronchial wash on bronchoalveolar lavage, or
        - Positive histopathology

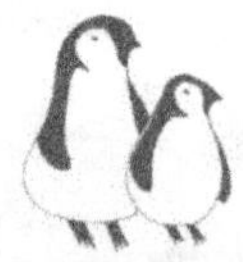

IGRA Interferon-γ Release Assays

- Release of interferon-γ from T cells indicates sensitization to M. tuberculosis
- More specific than TST, so is preferred for
  - Persons previously recovery PPD
  - Follow-up for persons who failed to report for a second visit to have their TST read

Bacteriology Testing

- Neither the finding of AFB (acid-fast bacilli) on a smear or the finding of caseating granulomas on histopathology are positive for active infection.
- Culture
  - Perform regardless of results of AFB smears
  - Time for results
  - NAA (nucleic acid amplification)
    - PPV > 95% when AFB smear is positive
    - When AFB smear is negative, but culture is positive, NAA is positive in 50% to 80%)

Cerebrospinal Fluid (CSF)

- AFB stains or cultures negative in 25% of TB meningitis
- Lymphocytic pleocytosis
- ↓ glucose, ↑ protein
- PCR
  - Sensitivity 50%
  - Specificity 98%

Chest X-Ray

- Give the characteristic changes on chest x-ray in TB, and from the findings, speculate what is the likely type of TB, and whether there is an increased pre-test probability of an associated risk factor.

Primary progressive	- Local infiltrates - Lymphadenophathy ▪ Hilar ▪ Paratracheal
Reactivation	- Fibrocavity superior segment of lower lobe - Apical posterior segment, upper lobes
HIV association	- Miliary pattern - Middle, lower lobe - Nodes near mediastinum - Pleural disease

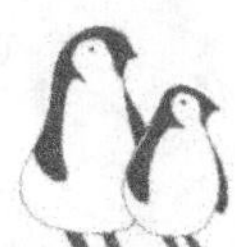

- Active TB
  - INH (plus pyridoxine), rifampin; ethamputol plus pyrazinamide for 2 mon
  - If this quadrupole program is interrupted for ≥ 2 wk, repeat course
- Maintenance (continuation) phase
  - INH (pyridoxine) plus rifampin
  - Duration, usual 4 mon
  - Special conditions, 7 mon

➢ Prevention
- Primary
  - BCG (Bacillus Calmette-Guerin) vaccination of children to prevent
    - Disseminated TB
    - TB meningitis
    - Avoid in persons with immunosuppression, since BCG is a live bacillus and vaccination would lead to widespread TB
  - Isolate and treat persons with acute TB
- Secondary
  - Treat LTBI

SO YOU WANT TO BE A PULMONARY PHYSICIAN!

TB can cause many different changes in the chest x-ray.

- Give the radiological findings on chest X-ray which suggest the type/ stage of the pulmonary TB.
  - Site
    - Lobe Upper (A-P segments)
      Lower (superior segments)
    - Hilum (lymphadenopathy)
  - Cavities
  - Infiltrate
    - Diffuse
    - Reticulonodular, uniform
      - Atypical/no findings
  - Type of TB
    - Primary progressive
    - Reactivation
    - Immunocompromised person with TB
    - Miliary

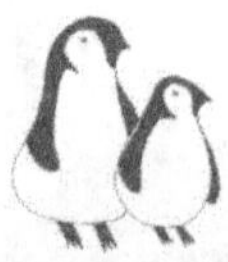

Three Tricks to Treat TB

- Give the general principles of treating TB in the setting of HIV co-infection.
  - As with all TB patients, do not use live vaccines, test for and if positive treat HBV / HCV, and do not use anti-TNF drugs
  - Begin anti-B therapy before anti-HIV therapy (ART, anti-retroviral therapy)
  - Same regimen and duration as non-HIV co-infection
  - Because of rifampin inducing cytochrome P450, the doses of ART may need to be increased
  - Pretreatment blood work/eye testing CBC complete blood count (for platelets)
    - LE (liver enzymes)
    - Creatinine
    - Visual
    - Acuity
    - Colour vision
  - Monitor for possible MDR (multidrug-resistant) strains of TB and XDR (extensively drug resistant)

- Give the meaning of MDR and XDR, and the implication to TB-infected persons.
  - MDR, resistance to INH, rifampin
  - XDR, resistance to INH, rifampin and fluoroquinolones, as well as 1 of the following
    - Kanamycin
    - Capromycin
    - Amikacin
  - Use more anti-TB medications for longer

- Give 5 characteristics of persons who are at ↑ risk of MDR and XDR.
  - Lack of response to appropriate regimen in an adherent patient
  - Previous TB treatment
  - Previous incorrect/inappropriate TB treatment
  - Poor patient adherence to treatment regimen
  - Infection with resistant strain possible
    - Country of origin
    - HIV-association
  - Close contact with other patients with resistant TB

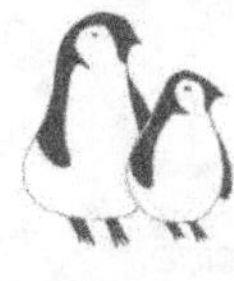

Four More Tricks to Treat TB

- Give the special condition when INH plus rifampin are given continuously for 7 rather than the usual 4 mon maintenance for active TB.
    - At diagnosis
        - Cavitary pulmonary TB, plus
        - At end of 4 mon maintenance, sputum cell culture still positive

- Give the duration of treatment of TB meningitis.
    - 9-12 mon of INH plus rifampin (plus an initial course of corticosteroids)

- It is often warned that corticosteroids should not be given to persons with TB. Give examples of when steroids are given with anti-TB drugs in order to enhance their effect.
    - TB meningitis
    - TB pericarditis
    - MAC (mycobacterium complex infection) pneumonitis

For more information on the use and adverse effects of fist- and second- line anti-tuberculosis drugs, please see a standard medical textbook, or a recent review such as UptoDate or MKSAP 16, Infectious disease 2012, Table 23, page 35.

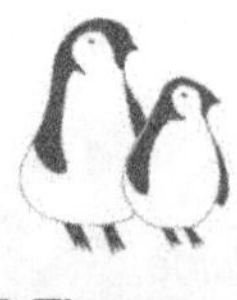

SO YOU WANT TO BE A PULMONOLOGIST!

- Give the name of 3 conditions causing both acute glomerulonephritis plus bleeding into the lungs (**pulmonary-renal syndrome**).
    - Wegner granulomatosis (aka granulomatosis with angiitis)
    - Anti-GBM (glomerular basement membrane) disease (aka Goodpasturedisease)
    - SLE (systemic lupus erythematosus)
    - Immune-complex mediated disorder

Non-Tuberculous Myobacteria (NTM)

- Source
    - Soil
    - Water
    - Medical equipment
- Demography
    - Young or older adults
    - Postmenopausal women
- Associated conditions

Lung (structural lung disease)	– COPD – Bronchiectasis – Cystic fibrosis (CF) – Pneumoconiosis
Esophagus	– Esophageal motility disorders
Heart	– MVP (mitral valve prolapse)
MSK	– Slim – Pectus excavatum – Scoliosis

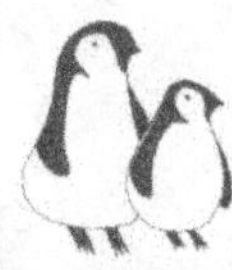

- Genetic defects in pathways for
  - Interferon-α
  - IL (interleukin)-12

- Diagnosis
  - Lung
    - Symptoms
    - Nodular or cavity disease on chest X-ray
  - Microbiology/ histology
    - Positive cultures
      - Sputum x2, or
      - Bronchoalveolar lavage x1, or
      - Positive NTM culute plus AFB and/or granulomas in tissue

Note:
- A common NTM is MAC (mycobacterium avium complex)
- For detained diagnostic criteria for NTM lung disease, please refer to a standard medical textbook or a recent review such as UptoDate or MKSAP 16, Infectious disease 2012, Table 25, page 37.

Mycobacterium Avium Complex Infection

- Sources
  - Inhaling aerosolized mycobacterium from water or soil
- Type
  - Fibrocavitary
  - Nodular bronchiectatic disease
    - Middle aged males or females who don't smoke and who don't have chronic lung disease
  - Disseminated HIV co-infection, CD4 < 50 / mL

  Note: MAC in children usually causes head and neck lymphangitis

- Treatment
  - Mild
    - Clarithromycin or azithromycin plus ethambutol plus rifampin or rifabutin
  - Severe
    - AS for mild (macrolide, ethambutol plus a rifamycin plus streptomycin or amikacin for the initial 1-2 mon
  - Corticosteroids for MAC pneumonitis
  - For lymphadenitis
    - Surgical exersion
  - Corticosteroids for MAC pneumonitis
  - For lymphadenitits
    - Surgical exersion

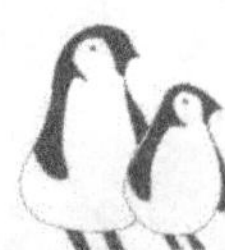

Rapidly Growing Mycobacterium (RGM)

- Saprophytes
- Direct inoculation or from water-contaminated medical equipment
- Sites of involvement
  - SSTI (skin and soft tissue)
  - Lung
  - MSK (muscoloskeletal)
- Multiple antibiotics regimen based upon in vitro susceptibility

Pneumocystis Jirovecii Pneumonia

- Cysts from sputum or bronchoscopy stain positive with silver stain.

- Give the range of changes on chest X-ray which suggest Pneumocystis Jirovecii Pneumonia.
  - Normal/non-specific
  - Diffuse infiltration
  - Consolidation
  - Pneumothorax
  - High index of suspicion in HIV patient with CD4 < 200 /μL (CT scan of chest may be useful)

➢ Prophylaxis

- Oral trimethoprim-sulfamethoxazole (TMS) when CD4 < 200 /μL

➢ Treatment

- Based on A-a, alveolar-arterial O_2 gradient, and PO_2
- 3 wk course
- No sulfa allergy

Severity	A-a mm Hg	Arterial PO_2 mm Hg	Rx
Mild	< 35	> 70	po TMS
Moderate	35-45	> 70	IV TMS plus
Severe	> 45	< 70	steroids

- Sulfa allergy
  - IV pentamidine, or
  - IV clindamycin, plus
  - PO primaquine

  plus corticosteriods based on A-a ≥ 35 mm Hg or arterial Po_2 < 70 mm Hg

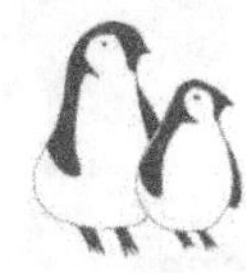

PULMONARY FUNGAL INFECTIONS

To be considered:

- Candidiasis
- Aspergillosis and Asperpilloma
- Mucormycosis
- Cryptococcus
- Blastomycosis
- Histoplasmosis
- Coccidiomycosis

Systemic/Invasive Candidiasis (C. albicans)

- Types of infection
  - Candidemia
  - Disseminate candidiasis
  - Focal organ involvement
  - Hepatosplenic (chronic disseminated)
- Risk factors
- Give risk factors for the development of candidiasis.
  - Drugs
    - Antibiotics, broad spectrum
    - Chemotherapy
    - Immunosuppressives
  - Catheters
    - TPN
    - Hemodialysis
  - Hospitalizations
  - Pancreatitis
  - Malignancy
  - Transplantation
  - Recent surgery
  - AKI (acute kidney injury)
  - Neutropenia

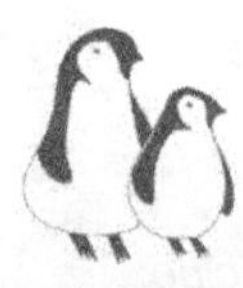

- Clinical microabscesses in virtually any organ but especially
  - Eye – White exudates
  - Skin – Painless papules/pustules on red base
  - MSK – Bone
    – Joints
  - GI – Peritoneum
  - GU – UTI

- Diagnosis
  - Culture
    - Blood "gold standard"
    - Negative blood culture does not exclude systemic candidiasis
    - Positive culture from any normally sterile area
    - "Candidiasis species that is obtained from a blood culture should never be considered a contaminant but instead should initiate investigation for a course" (MKSAP 16, Infectious disease 2012, page 39).
  - Tissue from skin lesion, or any involved organ

  Note: Since candida pneumonia is very rare, sputum culture if usually not done.

- Treatment
  - Non-neutropenic
    - Fluconazole
      - First choice for C. parapsilosis
      - If no/poor response, switch to
    - Echinocandin
      - Caspofungin
      - Anidulafungin
      - Micafungin
      - If echinocandin used first for empiric therapy and response is poor, may switch to Fluconazole if patient is stable
      - First choice empiric therapy for Candida glabrata
    - If echinocandin fails when used for C. glabrata, perform susceptibility testing before using
      - Fluconazole, or step-down
      - Voriconazole

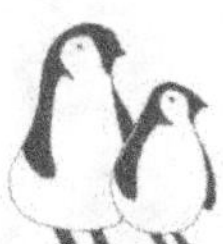

- Treat for 2 weeks after
  - Loss of symptoms
  - Clearance of fungemia
- Remove possibly causative catheters, central lines

- Neutropenic
  - Echinocandin, or
  - Voriconazole, or
  - Amphotericin B, echinocandin, or
  - Voriconazole
- Asymptomatic cystitis
  - Treat with fluconazole, if patient
    - Neutropenic
    - Having urologic surgery
- Focal infections
  - Meningitis
  - Endophthalmitis
  - Do not use echinocandins

Aspergillosis

- Cause
  - Inhalation of aerosolized spores of Aspergillus spores

- Types of pulmonary infection

Allergic bronchopulmonary aspergillosis	- Usually occurs in persons with ▪ Asthma ▪ Cystic fibrosis - Diagnosis ▪ Symptoms suggested of asthma ▪ Chest X-ray infiltations ("fleeting"), bronchiectasis, central ▪ Lab – ↑ eosinophils – ↑ serum IgE – Antibodies to Aspergillus ▪ Skin test – Reactivity to Aspergillus antigens - Treatment ▪ Itraconazole plus coticosteroids

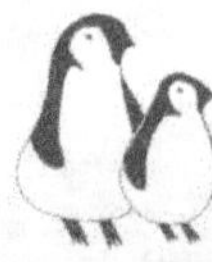

- Aspergilloma
  - Fungus ball in
    - A previous cyst/cavity
    - An area of dead (devitalized) lung
  - Positive sputum culture
  - Surgical resection

- Invasive/disseminated
  - Usually seen in immuncompromised persons
  - May involve lung, brain, other tissues

- Diagnosis

  - Chest X-ray
    - Infiltrates
    - Nodules
    - Infarcts

  - CT chest
    - Halo appearance necrotic area, surrounded by blood
    - Low attention around a nodule
    - Bleeding into tissue around the fungal infection
    - Caused by any type of angioinvasive fungi

  - Laboratory
    - Galactomannan antigen immunoassay
      - Serum
      - CSF
      - Bronchoalveolar lavage
    - B-D-glucan assay
    - PCR assay
    - Culture or histopathology is positive
    - Transthoracis percutaneous needle aspiration

- Treatment

  - Voriconazole

  - Salvage after voriconazole failure
    - Amphotericin B
      - Itraconazole
      - Posaconazole
    - Echinocandin
      - Caspofungin
      - Micafungin

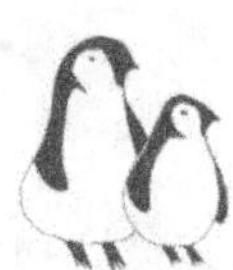

Mucormycosis

- Associated with
  - Immunosuppression
  - Neutropenia
  - Burns
  - Trauma
  - Diabetes
  - Drug
    - Corticosteroids
    - Chemotherapy
    - Deferoxamine
- Clinical
  - Mucormycosis may be suspected in the patient with
    - Sinusitis
    - Rhino-orbital infection
    - Rhino-cerebral infection
  - Commonest site of involvement overall: Rhinocerebral black necrotic material in nose and mouth
  - Commonest site with hematological malignancy pulmonary infarction from thrombosis
- Diagnosis
  - Tissue culture
  - Biopsy
    - "Broad, irregular, ribbon-like, aseptate hyphae"
  - Blood cultures
    - Usually negative

(MKSAP 16, Infectious disease 2012, page 14)

- Treatment
  - Urgent early and wide surgical debridement, plus
  - Amphoteracin B

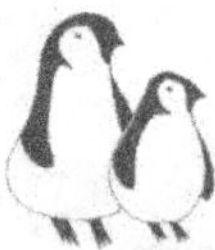

Cryptococcosis

- Clinical
  - Cryptococcus enters body though lungs and becomes disseminated in immunosuppressed persons
  - Commonest site of dissemination is CNS subacute/chronic meningitis meningoencephalitis
  - CNS complications are numerous
    - Brainstem vasculitis
    - Optic nerve involvement
    - Mass lesions
  - Note: "Whenever Cryptococcus occurs at a site outside CNS, a lumbar puncture should be done to determine if CNS infection is also present.
- Diagnosis
  - Cryptococcus antigen in serum or CSF
  - Positive culture or histopathology
- Therapy
  - For all CNS or extrapulmonary disease
  - Localized
    - Fluconazole
  - Disseminated
    - Induction therapy with amphotericin B plus flucytosine for 2-4 wk, then
    - Consolidation fluconazole for 8 wk
    - Maintenance
      - HIV-positive patient for 1 yr then stop if anti-viral therapy given and CD4 > 100 / mL for ≥ 3 mon
      - Organ transplant for life
  - Evidence of ↑ IC (intracranial pressure)
    - Removal of CSF by LP (lumbar puncture)
    - Ventriculoperitoneal shunt

CLINICAL CHALLENGE

A patient with HIV / AIDs presents with molluscam-like skin lesions and symptoms/signs of meningoencephalitis. Cryptococcosis is diagnosed.

- Give the therapy for disseminated cryptococcosis.
  - Normal renal function
    - Conventional formulation of amphotericin B plus flucytosine for 2 wk, followed by consolidation and maintenance (suppression) of cyptococcal infection for at least 8 wk.
  - Impaired renal function
    - Amphotericin B as a lipid formulation, plus flucytosine

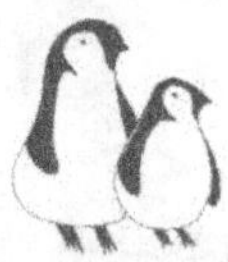

Blastomycosis

- Definition
  - "……… a systemic pyogranulomatous disease caused by Blastomyces dermatitides, a thermal dimorphic fungus that is endemic to states that border the Ohio and Mississippi river valleys as well as, states and Canadian provinces that border the Great Lakes and St. Lawrence River" (MKSAP 16, Infectious disease 2012, page 41)
- Commonest sites of involvement
  - Lung
  - Skin
- Diagnosis
  - Culture
  - Histopathology
- Treatment (pulmonary and extrapulmonary disease)
  - Mild
    - Itraconazole po for -12 mon
  - Severe
    - Amphotericin B for 1-2 wk, then
    - Itraconazole po for 6-12 mon

Histoplasmosis

- Cause
  - Histoplasma capsulatum, a thermal dimorphic fungus endemic to the Ohio and Mississippi river valleys, often an asymptomatic infection, but also causing
- Sites of disease
  - Lung
    - Pulmonary disease, acute and chronic
    - Bronchalithiasis
    - Histoplasmomas (nodules)
    - Cavitation
  - Mediastinum
    - Mediastinitis
      - Granulomatous
      - Fibrosing
    - Disseminated disease
- Treatment
  - Mild/moderate: Itraconazole
  - Severe: Amphotericin B

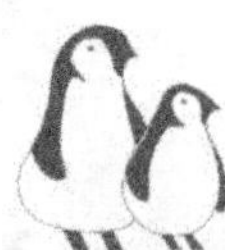

Coccidioidomycosis

- Cause
  - Inhalation of Coccidioidomycosis immitis and C. posaclasie thermal dimorphic fungus spores, endemic to deserts of Southwestern USA, Mexico, Central America
- Clinical
  - Acute-pneumonia-like illness
  - Subacute
    - Fever, respiratory symptoms, EN (erythema nodosum) skin rash
  - Extrapulmonary
    - Meningitis
    - Bones/joints
- Diagnosis
  - Serology
    - Serology, repeat testing
  - CSF
    - In presence of meningitis, may be negative
- Treatment
  - Mild/moderate
  - Severe
    - Including meningitis
      - Fluconazole po for life
    - Poor response to fluconazole Amphotericin B
    - Pregnant women for 3 to 6 mon (intrathecal)

Sporotrichosis

- Cause
  - Skin exposure soil containing Sporothrix schenckii→ ulcerating papule → lymphatic spread to bone/joints
- Diagnosis
  - Culture
- Treatment
  - Itraconazole

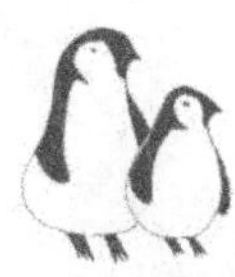

AIRFLOW OBSTRUCTION AND ASTHMA

Name Change: The postnasal drip syndrome is now called UACS (upper airway cough syndrome.

Asthma Syndromes

- Definition
  - "Asthma is a respiratory disorder characterized by
  - Paroxysmal or persistent [respiratory] symptoms
    - Dyspnea
    - Chest tightness
    - Wheezing
    - Sputum
    - Cough
  - Variable airflow limitation
  - Airway inflammation
  - Airway hyper-responsiveness

Source: Mc Cormack DG, et al. Chapter 51. In: Therapeutic Choices. Grey J, Ed. 6th Edition, *Canadian Pharmacists Association*: Otttawa, ON, 2011, page 671

- Differential: "All that 'wheeze' is not asthma
  - Wheezing
    - Wheezing on maximal forced exhalation
      - A sensitivity of only 57% and a specificity of only 37% for airflow obstruction.
      - A forced expiratory maneuver aimed at "unmasking silent bronchospasm" should not be relied on for the clinical diagnosis of airflow obstruction.
    - Wheezing that occurs only in exhalation
      - Not as severe as wheezing that occurs both in exhalation and inspiration.
      - Longer expiratory wheezes reflect worse obstruction than shorter expiratory wheezes.
    - Wheezes are not perfect diagnostic findings, and are less valuable than crackles.

Source: Mangione S. *Hanley & Belfus* 2000, page 327.

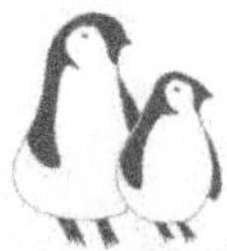

SO YOU WANT TO BE A RESPIROLOGIST!

- In the context of the patient with asthma, give the meaning of is the "**Loeffler syndrome**"?
    - Loeffler syndrome is comprised of
        - Asthma (airway reactivity)
        - Fever
        - Eosinophilia
        - Abnormal chest X-ray (transient, migratory pneumonitis; remember that persons with uncomplicated asthma will have a normal chest X-ray
    - Loeffler syndrome may be associated with
        - Polyartheritis
        - Allergic asthma
        - Allergic skin disease
        - Infections: mycoses, parasites
        - Drugs (e.g., Sulfa's, penicillin)
- How can you differentiate between chronic bronchitis or asthma versus emphysema by listening to the patient's breath sounds heard at the mouth (BSM) with the unaided ear, i.e., without using a stethoscope?
    - In chronic bronchitis and asthma, there is a positive relation between the loudness of BSM and the FEV_1, or PEFR (peaked expiratory flow rate), whereas in asthma, BSM, becomes softer as airflow obstruction worsens. Thus, the intensity of BSM is not increased in all persons with COPD.

Source: Mangione S. *Hanley & Belfus* 2000, page 304.

➢ Distinguish from other causes of widespread narrowing of airways resulting in wheezing

- Lung
    - COPD
    - PE
    - Tumour
- Heart
    - L-HF
- Immune
    - ELD
    - PAN

Abbreviation: ELD, eosinophilic lung disease; L-HF, left-sided heart failure; PAN, polyarteritis nodosum; PE pulmonary embolus; PHT, pulmonary hypertension; PR, pulse rate; RR, respiratory rate; SBP, systolic blood pressure

- Give the performance characteristics of pulsus paradoxus predicting severe asthma.

Finding	Sensitivity (%)	Specificity (%)	PLR	NLR
o 10 mm Hg	52-68	69-92	2.7	0.5
o 20 mm Hg	19-39	91-100	8.2	0.8
o 25 mm Hg	16	99	22.6	0.8

Abbreviations: NLR, negative likelihood ratio; PLR, positive predictive ratio

Source: McGee SR. *Saunders/Elsevier* 2007, Box 13.2, page 131.

➢ Differential diagnosis
  - o Larynx
    - Laryngeal edema
    - Laryngo-, trachea-, or bronchomalacia
    - Vocal cord dysfunction
  - o Trachea
    - Stenosis or compression
    - Foreign body
    - Central airway tumours
    - Aspiration
    - Vascular ring affecting trachea
  - o Heart
    - Heart failure
  - o Lung
    - Chronic obstructive pulmonary disease
    - Bronchorrheal states (such as chronic bronchitis, cystic fibrosis, bronchiectasis)
    - Hypersensitivity pneumonitis
    - Pulmonary edema
    - Forced expiration in normal subjects
    - Pulmonary embolism
    - Carcinoid syndrome
    - Löffler syndrome

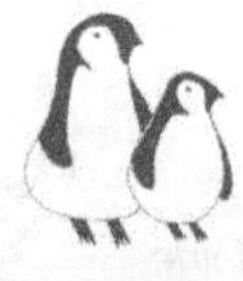

- Bronchiectasis
- Tropical eosinophilia
- α-1 Antiprotease deficiency
- Immotile cilia syndrome
- Bronchopulmonary dysplasia
- Bronchiolitis (including bronchiolitis obliterans), croup
- Cystic fibrosis
- Infections (croup, whooping cough, laryngitis, tracheobronchitis)

o Ribs
- Chondromalacia/polychondritis

o CNS
- Hyperventilation syndrome
- Facitious (including psychophysiological vocal cord adduction)

Adapted from: Ghosh AK. *Mayo Clinic Scientific Press* 2008, Table 2-5, 15.

Sweet Nothing: Not all that wheezes is "asthma".

➢ Clinical

- Give clinical syndromes which represent variants of asthma.

  - Occupational
  - Reactive airways dysfunction
  - Virus-induced
  - Cough-associated
  - GERD-associated
  - Allergic bronchopulmonary aspergillosis
  - Exercise-induced
  - Vocal cord dysfunction
  - Aspirin-sensitive

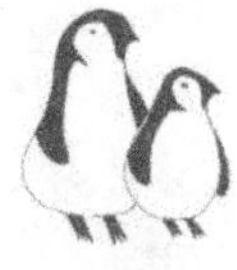

Occupational Asthma

- About 50% have late response (3-8 hr) after exposure to trigger
- Airway hyperresponsiveness may persist, so symptoms may persist even when away from occupational trigger
- Perform spirometry or determination of peak flow rate in and away from work environment
- Also perform
  - Bronchial challenge test
  - Skin testing, where possible
- Some reversibility of impaired lung function may occur over time when person away from adverse environment

Reactive Airways Dysfunction Syndrome (RADS)

- Rapid onset of symptoms shortly after single exposure to occupational irritant, without usual "allergic sensitization" which occurs with usual occupational asthma
- Even after single exposure to (NH3, choline, bleach), RADS symptoms may persist for years
- Diagnostic tests
  - Spirometry may be normal or abnormal
  - Bronchial challenge test positive

Virus-Induced Asthma

- Viruses which affect especially the upper airway may worsen asthma to joint of loss of asthma control, with need for intensification of therapy and even the need for hospitalization
- For up to 6 wk after a viral infection airway hyperresponsiveness may persist

Cough-Variant Asthma

- Dry cough rather than wheezing may be the only symptom
- It is important to include asthma in the differential of chronic cough, so that spirometry will be done to confirm the diagnosis and lead to proper therapy

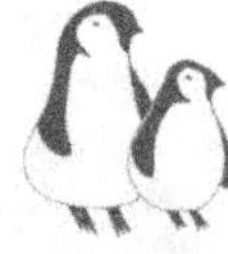

GERD-Associated Asthma

- Treatment with bid PPI for 3 mon may improve the symptoms of asthma in persons with symptomatic GERD
- In some cases a 24-hr esophageal pH study may be necessary to prove acid reflux, and to associated reflex events with the wheezing and other symptoms of asthma
- Exercise may ↑ microaspiration from GERD, and mimic exercise-induced bronchospasm (EIB)
- May be associated with VCD (vocal cord dysfunction)

Allergic Bronchopulmonary Aspergillosis (ABPA)

- Pathogenesis
  - Colonization of airways with the fungus Aspergillus famigatus leads to sensitization, inflammation, fibrosis and bronchiectasis
- Diagnosis
  - ↑ serum IgE, both ↑ total IgE and ↑ Aspergillus IgE
  - Eosinophilia
  - Positive skin test
  - Bronchiectasis in proximal airways from mucus plugs → atelectasis
  - Aggressive treatment with systemic corticosteroids needed to prevent pulmonary fibrosis

Vocal Cord Dysfunction

- Clinical

	Vocal Cord Dysfunction	Typical asthma
Onset/offset	Sudden	Slow
Wheeze	Inspiration (actually not wheeze, but stridor)	Expiration
Character of wheeze	Monophasic	Polyphonic
Localization	Neck	Chest
Associated with GERD	Yes	Yes

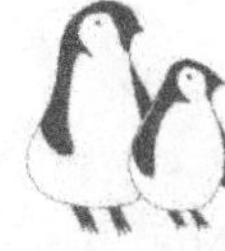

- Diagnosis

- Give the diagnosis findings of VCD (vocal cord dysfunction) on flow-volume loop testing, and on laryngoscopy.

  - Flow-loop testing
    - ↓ PEF
    - ↓ IF
    - Concave curve of PEF
  - Laryngoscopy
    - Adduction of vocal cords
    - ↓↓ size of opening in glottis

- Treatment
  - Acute episodes
    - Inhale helium-O_2 mixture, or
    - CPAP (continuous positive airway pressure)
  - Chronic maintenance
    - Behaviour modification
    - Speech therapy
  - Treat associated symptoms of GERD (gastroesophageal symptoms)

Aspirin-Sensitive Asthma

- Clinical
  - Suspect in difficult-to-control severe asthma, with associated link between symptoms and ASA (aspirin) intake, or intake of other drugs such as NSAIDs which ↑ leukotriene concentrations.

- In the context of aspirin-sensitive asthma, give the features of the **Samter triad**.

  - Samter triad is comprised of
    - Severe asthma
    - ASA sensitivity
    - Nasal polyps

- Treatment
  - Desensitization to ASA, with continued intake of ASA
  - Avoid NSAIDs

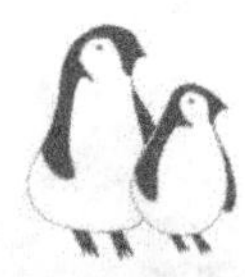

Exercise-Induced Bronchospasm (EIB) **Asthma**

- Persons with asthma often have ↑ bronchospasm with exercise (EIB, exercise-induced bronchospasm), especially when exercise undertaken in cold, dry air
- ↓ FEV1 ≥ 15% within 5-10 min after exercise
- The symptoms are worse after exercise has stopped
- Note that exercise may ↑ GERD, with microaspiration and bronchospasm
- Prevent EIB by inhaling B2-agonist 15 min before starting exercise, as well as warm-ups and wearing a cold weather mask

➢ Pathogenesis

- Reversible (airway obstruction)
- Bronchospasm
- Inflammation of airways
  - Infiltration
    - Eosinophils
    - Mast cells
    - Lymphocytes
    - Polymorphonuclear cells; neutrophils (PMNs)
- ~ 75% have identified allergies
- ↑ allergic inflammation (Th2 > Th1 response)
- Allergen
  - Early response (15-30 min) → mediators
    - Histamine
    - Leukotrienes
    - Tryptase
  - Late response (3-8 hr) → proinflammatory cytokines
- Repeated inflammation → remodeling, causing structural damage
  - Elastic fibers - Disruption
  - Subepithelium - Fibrosis
  - Mucus glands - Hyperplasia
  - Smooth muscle - Hyperplasia
- Eventual ↓ lung function

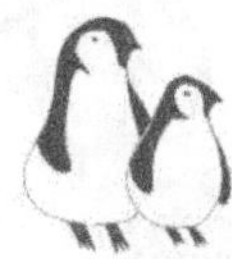

➢ Differential

- Consider alternate diagnosis if "asthma" is difficult to control

o Upper airways	– Obstruction
o Vocal cords	– Dysfunction
o Esophagus	– GERD (gastroesophageal reflux disease)
o Heart	– HF (heart failure)
o Lung	– COPD (chronic obstructive pulmonary disease) – Eosinophilic/allergic disorders

Finding	CEP	ABA	CSS
o Eosinophils	↑ serum	↑ serum	↑ biopsy
o Brown sputum	-	+	-
o Chest X-ray	Peripheral pulmonary edema	Intermittent infiltrates	Sinus and upper airway disease
o sIgE	-	↑	-
o Antibodies IgG / IgE	-	+	-
o pANCA to Aspergillus	-	+	-
o Skin test	-	+	-

Abbreviation: ABA, allergic bronchopulmonary aspergilosis; CEP, chronic eosinophilic pneumonia; CSS, Churg-Straus syndrome

➢ Clinical

- Take a directed history for asthma.
  - Wheezing
    - Acute/chronic (duration)
    - Onset/offset
    - Cough/wheeze recurrent
      - Worse at night emotion, or after exercise
      - Improvement with bronchodilators
    - Fever, chills
    - Aspiration
    - Cardiac disease
    - Personal history of eczema, hay fever
    - Immunizations

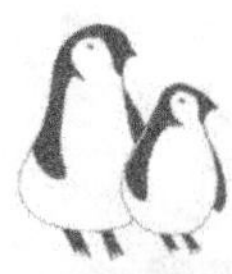

- Family history of
- Past history
  - Atopy (hay fever, eczema)
  - Nasal polyps
  - Rhinitis
  - Asthma
  - Allergies
- Tightness of chest

- Associations
  - ENT
    - Sinusitis
    - Rhinitis
    - Vocal cord dysphonia
  - GI
    - GERD (gastroesophageal reflex disease)
  - CNS
    - OSA (obstructive sleep apnea)

- Complications
  - ER visits
  - Hospital admissions, ICU, intubation
  - Use of beta-blockers
  - Medications, including Tablets, inhalers, ASA, steroids

- Causes
  - Seasonal allergies – pollens, foods, animals, medications
  - Upper respiratory infection
  - Medications
  - Family history of other pulmonary conditions
  - Exercise
  - Cold weather
  - Smoke - first/second hand
  - Stress
  - Gastroesophageal reflux disease

Adapted from: Filate W, et al. *The Medical Society, Faculty of Medicine, University of Toronto* 2005, page 290; Jugovic PJ, et al. *Saunders/ Elsevier* 2004, page 107.

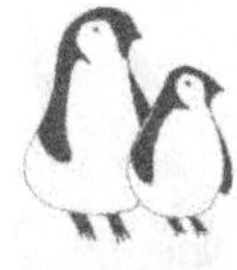

- Perform a focused physical examination of the patient with asthma.
  - Ability to speak (inability to complete a sentence in one breath)*
  - Restlessness
  - Altered mental status, confusion, coma*
  - Fatigue, exhaustion*
  - Vital signs (RR, HR, BP, O_2 saturation)
  - Wheezing
  - Dyspnea
  - Inspiration
    - ↑ use of accessory respiratory muscles
    - ↓ ability to speak
  - Auscultation
    - ↓ breath sounds
  - PFT
    - FEV1, PEF < 40% of predicted 1 hr often bronchodilators
  - Cardiology
    - PR> 110 bpm*
    - Pulsus paradoxus (not useful to predict severity of asthmatic attack)
    - Cyanosis
    - ↓ PR, ↓ BP*
  - Respiratory
    - RR >25/min*
    - ↓ RR (poor respiratory effort)*
    - Cyanosis*
    - Barrel chest
    - Cough
    - Sputum
    - Accessory muscle use
    - ↓ Air entry / silent chest
    - Wheezes and location (bilateral, scattered)
    - Crackles and location
    - Percussion – hypertympanic
    - Prolonged expiration
    - Clubbing
    - Peak expiratory flow rate less than 50% of predicted or best*
  - Signs of complications
    - PHT/ CHF (cor pulmonale)

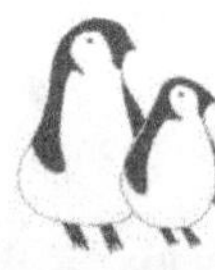

- Focus of infection
  - Rhinorrhea, coryza
  - Pharynx
  - Tympanic membrane
  - Cardiovascular examination
  - Abdominal examination
  - Skin examination – rash

*denotes severe asthmatic attack (risk stratification)

Adapted from: Jugovic PJ, et al. *Saunders/ Elsevier* 2004, page 108; McGee SR. *Saunders/Elsevier* 2007, page 338; Baliga RR. *Saunders/Elsevier* 2007, page 260.

- Remember

– Bilateral crackles	▪ HF (heart failure)
– Large volume of purulent sputum clubbing	▪ Bronchiectasis ▪ Cystic fibrosis
– ↑ IgE, eosinophilia	▪ Allergic bronchopulmonary aspergillosis

➢ Diagnosis

- History and physical
- Spirometry usually ↓ FEV1 / FVC, ≥ 12% better with bronchodilators
- Bronchial challenge test usually positive
  - Contraindicated in pregnancy
- Allergy skin testing, with assessment of clinical relevance
  - Not recommended in pregnancy
- Allergen-specific ↑ serum IgE concentrations
- Exhaled NO (nitric oxide) measurements (correlates with airway)
  - Inflammation
  - Eosinophilia

- Give the test which may be used to prove the asthmatic patient, claim that they have been adherent to their prescribed corticosteroids.
  - When the inflammation associated with asthma is reduced by corticosteroids, the baseline exhaled NO declines.

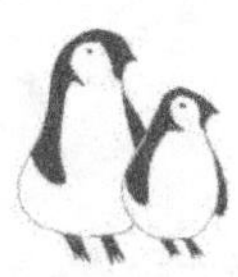

- Give the diagnostic tests which you will perform in patient with difficult to control symptoms of asthma, recurrent pulmonary infiltration, as well as signs of early brochectasis ABPA (allergic bronchopulmonary aspergillosis).
  - Skin test (high sensitivity, high negative predictive value)
  - IgE > 1000 IU/mL favors diagnosis; < 500 IU.mL disfavors diagnosis
  - Eosinophils (↑)
  - Precipitating antibodies to Aspergillus fumigatus

➤ Therapy (based on asthma step classification, which is based on frequency of worse feature of symptoms).

Clinical Scenarios

Guidelines recommend using long-acting β-agonists plus corticosteroids for moderate persistent asthma (need to use short-acting β-agonists daily, nocturnal symptoms ≥ 1 /wk, or acute exacerbations ≥ 2 /wk).

- Give the reason why long-acting β-agonists are not used without accompanying corticosteroids.
  - Long acting β-agonists used on their own actuality ↑ mortality

- In the patient with moderate persistent asthma in which the asthma may have been triggered by an infection, give the reason why the recommended treatment is
  - Long-acting β-agonist plus corticosteroid, or
  - Corticosteroid by itself, or
  - Corticosteroid plus leukotriene modifier

In other words, avoid using corticosteroid plus theophylline when the patient may require an antibiotic:

- The antibiotics which would usually be used for a pulmonary infection in association of a flare of asthma would include fluoroquinolones or macrolides.
- Fluoroquinolones or macrolides would ↑ theophylline concentration, possibly into the toxic range.

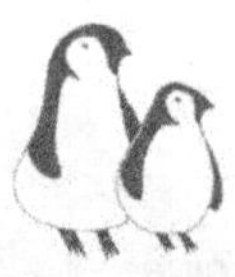

➢ Treatment

• Give the treatment of asthma.

Classification	Symptoms	Nocturnal Symptoms	Treatment
○ Intermittent	≤ 2 / wk	≤ 2 / mon	– β-agonist, short-acting, prn
○ Mild persistent	> 2 / wk but < 1 /d	> 2 / mon	- β-agonist, short-acting, plus inhaled corticosteroid, low-dose,
○ Moderate persistent	Need to use short-acting β-agonist daily	≥ 1 / wk, or acute exacerbations ≥ 2 / wk	– β-agonist, long-acting (salmeterol, or formoterol), plus corticosteroid, low-/medium-dose, inhaled or – Corticosteroid, inhaled medium dose, or – Corticosteroid, low-/medium-dose, plus inhaled theophylline or – Leukotriene modifier
○ Severe persistent	Continual symptoms that limit physical activity	"frequent"	– Corticosteroid, high-dose, inhaled, plus long-acting bronchodilator +/- corticosteroid, oral

○ Note
- Oral / IV corticosteroids e.g., prednisone 40 mg / day for 7 days may be needed for severe attack.

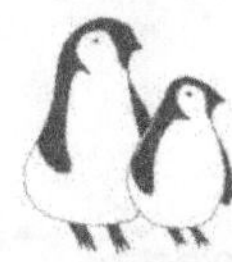

Classification	Treatment

o Severe exacerbations	- Hospitalization
	- Blood gas
	- Repeated doses albuterol
	  - Nebulizer, continuous flow, or
	  - Inhaler, metered-dose with spacer
	- IV corticosteroids, if albuterol not effective
	- Ipatropium, inhaled
	- IV magnesium sulfate

o Complications	- Related to use of corticosteroids
o Immunization	- Influenza - Pneumococcus

A patient with severe asthma does not respond satisfactorily to treatment with high dose inhaled corticosteroids and a long-acting β2-agonist.

- Give the criteria for using omalizumab.
  - o Severe asthma
    - Not responsive to usual therapy
    - History of allergies
    - ↑ IgE in serum

Severe exacerbations of asthma are routinely treated with supplemental O_2 IV corticosteroids, and inhaled anti-cholinergics and short-acting β2-agonists.

- Give adjunct interventions which may be useful, but which are not included in most interventional guidelines.
  - o Magnesium sulphate 2 g
    - IV, given once
  - o Inhalation of
    - Helium (60%) and oxygen (40%)
  - o Non-invasive ventilation

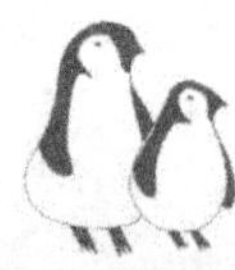

Clinical Alert

In the patient with a severe exacerbation of asthma if the arterial PCO_2 is normal, get ready to ventilate the patient since they are heading towards respiratory failure.

- Give the features on physical examination and chest X-ray which would increase the likelihood of **cystic fibrosis** in a young patient with asthma and a positive family history.
    - Digit clubbing
    - Nasal polys
    - Chest X-ray showing upper-lobe bronchiectasis

- Give factors which would raise the likelihood of vocal cord dysfunction (VCD).
    - History of acute onset and offset attacks
    - Discomfort in neck
    - Inspiratory plus expiratory wheezing
    - No hypoxemia
    - No hyperinflation on chest X-ray

Intermittent Asthma

➤ Definition
- Asthma symptoms ≤ 2 days / wk
- Use of short-acting β2-agonist (SABA) ≤ 2 days / wk [not including SABA use for EIB [exercise-induced bronchospasm])
- Nighttime awakening ≤ 2 times/month
- No interference with normal activity

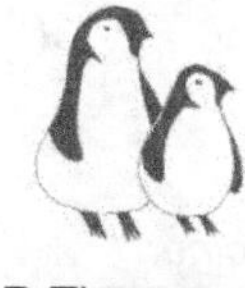

- Lung function
  - FEV1 normal between attacks. > 80% of predicted
  - FEV1 / FVC normal

➢ Treatment

- Remove offending agents
- Supplemental O_2 to keep saturation > 92%
- SABA (short-acting β2 agonists) prn (as needed ≤ 3 inhalations
- Inhalers
  - MDIs (metered-dose inhalers), +/- spacer at 20-min intervals
  - DPIs (dry powder inhalers)
- SABA may be used together with short-acting anti-cholinergic e.g., ipratropium

- Give a classification of severity of persistent asthma (based on clinical aspects and pulmonary function testing), and a step-up approach to pharmacological therapy.

	Clinical			Lung Testing	
Classification of Persistent Asthma	Symptoms, and Use of SABA to Relieve Symptoms	Nighttime Awakenings per Month	Limitation of Normal Physical Activity	FEV1, % of Predicted	FEV1 / FVC
o Mild	> 2 days / wk, but not daily	3-4	Mild	> 80	Normal
o Moderate	Daily	> 1 / wk	Moderate	> 60 < 80	↓ 5%
o Severe	Throughout the day	Nightly	Severe	< 60	↓ > 5%

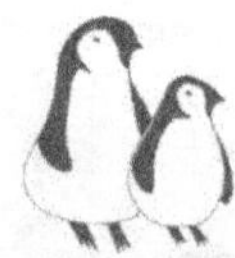

Therapy	2 PEFR 40 - 69%	3 PEFR < 40%	4	5	6
➢ Recommended					
o ICS (inhaled corticosteroid)	Low-dose	Low-dose	Medium-dose	High-dose	High-dose
o LABA (long-acting B2 agonist)	-	LABA*	LABA	LABA	LABA
o po CORT (oral corticosteroid)	-	- Or Medium-dose ICS but no LABA	-	-	po CORT
o OMAL (omalizumab)	-	Low-dose	Medium-dose		
➢ Alternate					
o ICS	-	-	-	OMAL**	OMAL
o LTRA (leukotriene receptor antagonist) / LPI (5-lipoxygenase inhibitor)	LTRA, LPI Or	LTRA, LPI Or	LTRA, LPI Or		
o Theophylline	THEO	THEO	THEO		

Modified from MKSAP 16 2013, Pulmonary, Table 4, page 13.

* Long-acting anti-cholinergic (LAACh), such as tiotropium may be considered in place of LABA. Also LTRA (leukotriene receptor antagonists), LPI (5-lipoxygenase inhibitors), and theophylline may be used in place of LABA

** For patients with severe asthma, bronchial thermoplasty (bronchoscope inserted catheter to give warm air connected to a radiofrequency generator) may be used for its modest short term benefit

When all else fails, immune modulation may need to be considered.
Note: Once asthma symptoms have been controlled for 3 months, consider reversing this step-up process.

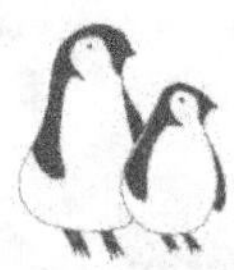

Classes of Asthma Medications

- β2-agonists
  - Short-acting
  - Long-acting
- Anti-cholinergics
- Corticosteroids
- Leukotriene receptor antagonists
- Theophylline
- Anti-IgE antibody

β2-agonists

➢ Short-acting	○ "reliever" of intermittent symptoms (≤ 2 days / wk) from - Allergens - Exercise - Cold/dry air ○ Examples: Albuterol, levalbuterol, metaproterenol, pirbuterol ○ Albuterol is safe for intermittent use in pregnancy
➢ Long-acting	○ "controller" of frequent symptoms (persistent asthma, Step 3, and above) ○ Added to ICS (inhaled corticosteroids) for symptom control ○ Must be used with agent to ↓ inflammation, such as ICS ○ Salmeterol, formoterol, 12 hr duration ○ Because of concern about ↑ morbidity/mortality from use of LABA (long-acting β-agonist), consider using long-acting anti-cholinergic tiotropium together with ICS

Safety alert re long-acting β2 agonist

- Long-acting β2 agonist
  - Used without ICS ↑ risk of asthma morbidity and mortality
  - Must not be used on their own

Note: The receptor function of β2-agonists is increased by corticosteroids, so there is ↑ effectiveness of the β2-agonists.

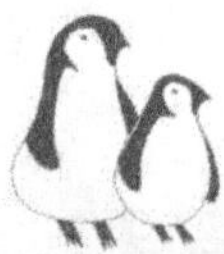

Anti-Cholinergic Agents

- Short-acting anti-cholinergic (SAAch), e.g., ipratropium
    - ↑ bronchodilation produced by SABA (short-acting beta agonist), and treatment may include SABA plus short-acting anti-cholinergic (SAAch, e.g., albuterol)
    - "reliever" or co-reliever of intermittent symptoms
- Long-acting
    - Tiotropium may be added to ICS for symptom control rather than LABA (long-acting β agonist)

Inhaled Corticosteroids (ICS)

- "controller" therapy for persistent asthma
- ↓ inflammatory cells numbers and activity
    - Mast cells
    - Eosinophils
    - Lymphocytes
- ↓ late-phase response to allergens
- ↑ function of receptors for β2-agonists → ↑ effect of β2-agonists
- In COPD
    - Do not use ICS as monotherapy
    - ICS does not reduce the progressive ↓ FEV1

Trick question

- Give the effect of ICS on neutrophils (PMN), number and activity of mast cells, eosinophils and lymphocytes, eosinophils and lymphocytes.
    - ICS → ↑ PMN
    - ↓ mast cells, eosinophils, lymphocytes

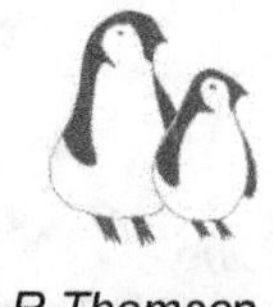

- Note:
  - ↑ risk of pneumonia (when used for COPD)
  - Given the life-saving nature of corticosteroids in patients with persistent asthma, the risk of adverse effects are considered to be "acceptable"
  - The locally acting budesonide has much fewer systemic effects as compared with the non-locally acting steroids

Leukotriene-Modifying Drugs

- Mechanisms of action
  - Montelukast, zafirlukast – LTRA (leukotriene receptor antagonists) inhibitors (LPI)
  - Zileuton – 5-lipoxygenase → ↓ production of leukotrienes

- Uses
  - LTRA / LPI may be alternative to LABA or ICS for combination of ICS + LTRA for persistent asthma, Step 3, and above.

- Give the major adverse effects (AEs) of the use of LTRA and LPI.
  - LTRA – Neuropsychological AEs, e.g.,
    - Agitation
    - Anxiety
    - Depression
    - Hallucinations
    - Thoughts of suicide
  - LPI – Hepatotoxicity

Methylxanthines

- Mechanism of action is unknown
- Narrow therapeutic margin to its relative weak bronchodilation
- Target concentration for monitoring theophylline
- Numerous drugs ↑ concentration of theophylline → ↑ risk of adverse effects (AEs)

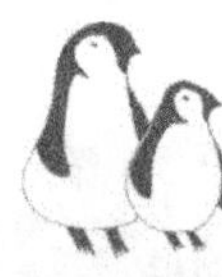

- Adverse effects (AEs)
  - CNS
    - Headache
    - Tremor
    - Seizure
  - GI
    - Nausea
  - CVS
    - Palpitations
    - Arrhythmias

Anti-IgE Antibody

- Omalizumab is a recombinant antibody which blocks the fragment crystallisable portion (Fc) of IgE, preventing the release of histamine and leukotrienes from mast cells and basophils.
- Consider for patients with
  - Persistent asthma
  - Step 5 to 6 in the stepwise approach to asthma therapy
  - IgE concentration
    - 30-700 kilounits / L
    - 30-700 IU / mL

Safety alert

- Omalizumab users have a risk of ~ 100 / 10^5 patients of severe anaphylaxis reactions, so users must be observed after each treatment.

Asthma in Pregnancy

- Give the care of asthma in the pregnant woman.
  - Diagnosis
    - Spirometry +/- bronchodilators
    - Do **not** perform
      - Bronchial challenge testing
        - **Contraindicated**
      - Skin testing
        - **Not** recommended

- Give 3 risks associated with poorly controlled asthma in pregnancy.
  - Mother
    - Preeclampsia
    - Premature labor
  - Child
    - ↓ birth weight
    - ↑ mortality rate

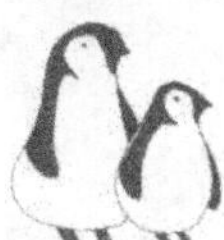

- Treatment
  - Regular monitoring
  - SABA (albuterol) plus ICS (especially locally acting budesonide)
  - Depending on severity, may use
    - LABA, long-acting beta agonist
    - LAAch, long-acting anti-cholinergic
    - LTRA, leukotriene receptor antagonist
    - LPI, 5-lipoxygenase inhibitor
    - THEO, theophylline

SPECTRUM OF OBSTRUCTIVE PULMONARY DISEASES

Bronchitis

- Definitions
  - Chronic bronchitis
    - Cough with mucoid expectoration for at least 3 months in a year for 2 successive years.
  - Emphysema
    - The abnormal permanent enlargement of the airway distal to the terminal respiratory bronchioles with destruction of their walls. (Clinical, radiological and lung function tests give an imprecise picture in an individual case, but a combination of all these features gives a reasonable picture)
  - The term COPD (chronic obstruction pulmonary disease) encompasses chronic obstructive bronchitis (with obstruction of small airways) and emphysema (with destruction of lung parenchyma, loss of lung elasticity, and closure of small airways).
    - Most patients also have mucus plugging

Source: Baliga RR. *Saunders/Elsevier* 2007, page 262.

- Take a focused history and perform a directed physical examination for chronic bronchitis.
  - General
    - Sputum cup full
    - Pursed lip
    - O_2 mask/respirator
    - Cyanosis of lips/tongue

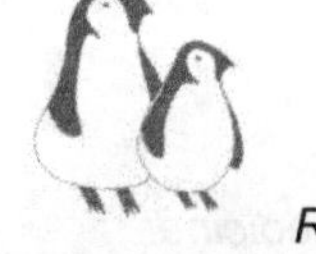

- Neck
  - Inspection
    - Use of accessory muscles of respiration (sternocleidomastoids, scaleni and trapezi)
    - ↑ JVP
  - Palpation
    - Tracheal deviation
    - ↓ distance (< 3 fingers' breadth) between the cricoid cartilage and suprasternal notch
- Lungs
  - Inspection
    - Barrel-shaped
    - ↑ RR
    - Dyspnea
    - Chest expansion
  - Palpation
    - Apex beat
    - ↓ Chest expansion
    - Tactile vocal fremitus
  - Percussion
    - Hyper-resonance
  - Auscultation
    - ↓ breath sounds
    - Vocal resonance
    - Forced expiratory time > 6 seconds indicates airflow obstruction
- CVS
  - ↑ PR
  - Bounding pulse
  - ↓ heart dullness
  - Displaced apex beat
  - ↑ P_2
- Abdomen
  - ↓ liver dullness
  - Palpable liver (not necessarily enlarged)
- Hands
  - Warm palms
  - Tar staining
  - No clubbing

Abbreviations: RR, respiratory rate; PR, pulse rate

Adapted from: Baliga RR. *Saunders/Elsevier* 2007, pages 261 and 262.

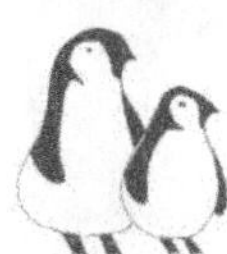

- Take a directed history to differentiate between bronchial asthma, chronic bronchitis, and emphysema.

Differential Feature	Bronchial Asthma	Chronic Bronchitis ("blue bloater")	Emphysema ("pink puffer")
Onset	70% < 30 y	>50 y	$\leq$ 60 y
Cigarette smoking	0	++++	++++
Pattern	Paroxysmal	Chronic, progressive	Chronic, progressive
Dyspnea	0 to ++++	+ to ++++	+++ to ++++
Cough	0 to +++	++ to ++++	+ to +++
Sputum	0 to ++	Profuse, mucopurulent	scanty
Atopy	50% (adult)	15%	15%
Infections	↑ Symptoms	↑↑↑ Symptoms	↑ Symptoms
Cyanosis	---	++	--
Hyperinflation	---	+	++
Cor Pulmonale	---	+++ frequent, remittent	+ (pre-terminal)
Respiratory drive	---	↓	↑
Polycythemia	---	+++	+
Chest X ray, vessels	---	---	↓
Arterial PCO_2	---	↑	
Alveolar gas transfer	---	---	↓

Adapted from: Ghosh, AK. *Mayo Clinic Internal Medicine Review.* 8th Edition. page 902; Baliga RR. *Saunders/Elsevier*, 2007, page 2; Burton JL. *Churchill Livingstone* 1971, page 26.

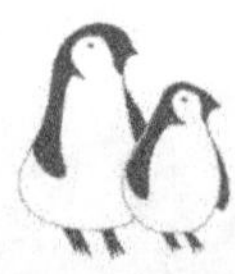

Useful background: Operational characteristics of clinical features in emergency department patients with history of asthma or COPD.

Finding	PLR	NLR
➢ Initial clinical judgment	9.9	0.65
➢ History		
o Atrial fibrillation	4.1	0.74
o Coronary artery bypass grafting	2.8	0.92
o Myocardial infarction	2.2	0.84
o Diabetes mellitus	2.0	0.85
o Coronary artery disease	2.0	0.67
➢ Physical examination		
o S3 (ventricular filling gallop)	57	0.83
o JVP	4.3	0.65
o Lower extremity edema	2.7	0.41
o Lung rales	2.6	0.39
o Hepatic congestion	2.4	0.91
➢ Chest radiograph		
o Edema	11	0.68
o Cardiomegaly	7.1	0.54
o Pleural effusion(s)	4.6	0.78
➢ Electrocardiogram		
o Atrial fibrillation	6.0	0.73
o Ischemic ST-T waves	4.6	0.83
o Q waves	3.1	0.84
o BNP$\geq$ 100 pg/mL	4.1	0.09

Abbreviations: BNP,brain natriuretic peptide; NLR, negative likelihood ratio, PLR, positive likelihood ratio

Note that some clinical features are not shown here because their likelihood ration is < 2. These include history of angina, hypertension, symptoms of orthopnea, fatigue, nocturnal cough, enlarged heart, wheezing, chest X-ray showing pneumonia, hyperinflation or normal.

Adapted from: Simel DL, et al. *JAMA* 2009, Table 16-9, page 203.

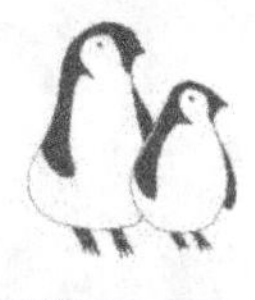

Chronic Obstructive Pulmonary (Lung) Disease (COPD)

- Definition
  - Slow progressive inflammation of the airways and lung parenchyma, leading to airflow obstruction (post-bronchodilator FEV1 / FVC <70%)

- Terminology
  - Chronic obstructive bronchitis
    - Productive cough for at least 3 months a year for 2 successive years
    - Obstruction of small airways
  - Emphysema
    - Abnormal, permanent dilation of the pulmonary airway distal to the terminal respiratory bronchioles destruction of the walls (↓ lung parenchyma)
    - ↓ lung elasticity
    - Closure of small airways
    - Mucus plugging
  - COPD
    - Includes chronic bronchitis and emphysema
  - Bronchiectasis
    - Chronic, necrotizing infection of bronchi and beonchioles
    - Abnormal, permanent dilation of airways

- Pathophysiology

Inflammation of small airways	- Narrowing ▪ Bronchiolitis → mucus plugs → fixed (non-reversible) obstruction ▪ Fibrosis → ↓ DLCO
Protease release	- ↓ elastic tissue ▪ ↓ recoil ▪ ↓ expiratory airflow ▪ ↑ duration of expiration ▪ ↑ RV ▪ ↑ EELV ▪ ↓ FVC - ↓ tissue adjacent to airways ▪ Emphysema ▪ ↓ capillaries - ↑ static hyperinflation → air trapping → dynamic hyperinflation

Abbreviation: DLCO, diffusion capacity for carbon monoxide; EELV, end-expiratory lung volume; FVC, forced vital capacity; RV, residual volume

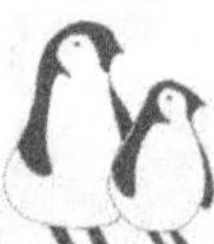

- Cause, associations and risk factors

o High level of heterogeneity of COPD	- Multiple genes
o Inherited, α1-AT (anti-trypsin deficiency)	- α1-antichymotrypsin - α2-amcroglobulin - Vitamin D binding protein - Blood group antigens
o Irritants	- Tobacco smoke - Smoke from biomass energy - Pollution
o Lung disease	- Asthma - Pulmonary TB (tuberculosis)

  - Socioeconomic challenge, malnutrition

Research agenda

- Only 20% of heavy smokers develop COPD. Why?
- About 20% of COPD patterns occur in non-ever-smokers. Why?

- Clinical
  - Great heterogeneity in type or severity of pulmonary or extrapulmonary clinical presentations
  - Pulmonary
    - Lung
      - Parenchyma
      - Pneumonia
        - Atelectasis
      - Airways
      - Pleura
        - Pneumothorax
      - Blood pressure
        - PHT (pulmonary hypertension)
    - Heart
      - Cor pulmonale

- Note: there are several means to assess severity of COPD.
    - MMRC (modified medical research Council Dyspnea Score)
    - GOLD (Global Institute for Chronic Obstructive Lung Disease)
    - BODE (BMI, obstruction, dyspnea, exercise), Index composite score
    - CAT (COPD assessment test)
        - Please see www.catestonline.org for details
    - Clinical COPD questionnaire
        - Please see www.ccq.nl for details

- Extrapulmonary associations

- CNS	▪ Depression ▪ CVA (cerebrovascular accident, aka stoke) ▪ OSA (obstructive sleep apnea)
- Eyes	▪ Glaucoma ▪ Cataracts
- ENT	▪ Sinusitis
- Endocrine	▪ Diabetes ▪ ED (erectile dysfunction)
- Bone	▪ Osteoporosis
- GI	▪ GERD (gastroesophageal reflux disease)
- CVS	▪ Hypertension ▪ Hypercholesterolemia ▪ CAD (coronary artery disease) ▪ HF (heart failure) ▪ AF (atrial fibrillation) ▪ Embolization
- MSK	▪ Arthralgias
- Cancer	

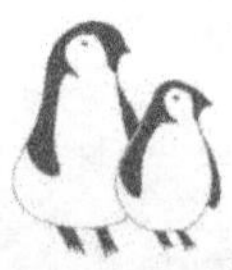

- Give the operating characteristics of clinical history for COPD.

Item	PLR	NLR
o Smoking history		
– ≥70 vs <70 pack yrs	8.0	0.63
o Sputum production ≥ ¼ cup	4	0.84
o Symptoms of chronic bronchitis	3.0	0.78
o Wheezing	3.8	0.66
o Exertional dyspnea		
- Grade 4 vs 3 or less	3.0	0.98
- Any vs none	2.2	0.83
o Wheezing	36	0.85
o Barrel chest	10	0.90
o Decreased cardiac dullness	10	0.88
o Match test	7.1	0.43
o Rhonchi	5.9	0.95
o Hyperresonance	4.8	0.73
o Forced expiratory time, sec		
>9	4.8	
6-9	2.7	
<6	0.45	
o Subxiphoid cardiac apical impulse	4.6	0.94
o Pulsus paradoxus (>15 mm Hg)	3.7	0.62
o Decreased breath sounds	3.7	0.70

Abbreviation: PLR, positive likelihood ratio; NLR negative likelihood ratio

Adapted from: Simel DL, et al. *JAMA* 2009 Chapter 13, Table 13-2, page 152, and Table 13-3, page 154.

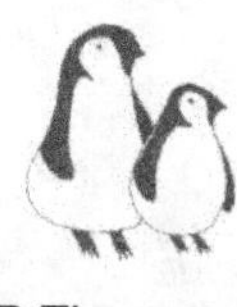

SO YOU WANT TO BE A RESPIROLOGIST!

- Is the Campbell sign specific for COPD?
  - Tracheal descent with inspiration ("tracheal tug", aka the Campbell sign) is caused by any cause of chronic airflow obstruction, and not just COPD.

Source: Mangione S. *Hanley & Belfus* 2000, page 287.

- Take a directed history for the harmful effects of cigarette smoking.
  - CNS
    - Autonomic: transient stimulation, followed by depression of all ganglia
    - CNS: stimulation, especially respiratory, vasomotor and emetic centres
    - Antidiuretic: (due to ADH release)
    - Tobacco amblyopia
  - CVS
    - Rise in BP, tachycardia, cutaneous vasoconstriction
    - Tobacco angina
    - Atrial extrasystoles
    - Myocardial ischemia
    - Buerger disease
  - Lung
    - Post-operative pneumonia
    - Bronchitis
    - Bronchus (increased carcinoma incidence)
  - GI
    - Esophagus (increased carcinoma incidence)
    - Cirrhosis incidence increased (probably due to associated alcoholism)
  - Kidney
    - Prostate (increased carcinoma incidence)
    - Bladder (increased carcinoma incidence)

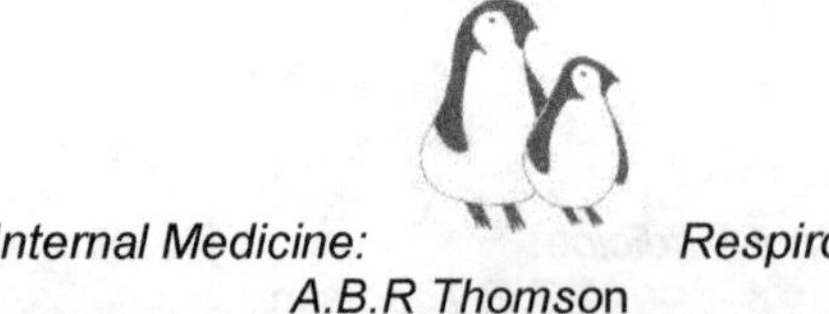

- Endocrine
  - Adrenal: discharges adrenaline
  - Hypoglycemia
- Fetus (pregnant mother smoking)
  - ↓ fetal growth
  - ↑perinatal mortality rate

Adapted from: Burton JL. *Churchill Livingstone* 1971, page 27.

➢ Risk stratification

- **Modified Medical Research Council** (MMRC) **Dyspnea Score for Severity of Dyspnea***

Severity	MMRC Score	Level of Shortness of Breath on Exertion
o None	0	– With strenuous exercise
o Mild	1	– Walking up slight hill
o Moderate	2	– Walking on level ground
o Severe	3	– Stop walking after 100 m
o Very severe	4	– Dyspnea on dressing/undressing

* For full details, please see MKSAP 16 2013, Pulmonary, Table 9, page 20.

- **Gold Composite Score**
  - Based on
    - Gold score
    - MMRC score
    - Exacerbations per year

Patient	Risk	Symptoms	Gold Stage	Exacerbations per Year	MMRC Score
A	Low	Few	1 or 2	≤ 1	< 2
B	Low	More	1 or 2	≤ 1	≥ 2
C	High	Few	3 or 4	≥ 2	< 2
D	High	More	3 or 4	≥ 2	≥ 2

Adapted from MKSAP 16 2013, Pulmonary, Table 10, page 20.

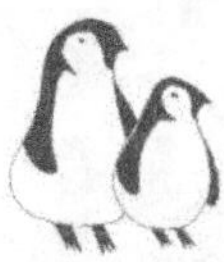

GOLD (Global Initiative for Chronic Obstructive Lung Disease) Stage for reduced airflow based on FEV1, after bronchodilator, in COPD patients with FEV1 / FVC < 70%.

Gold Classification	Clinical Description	FEV1, of Predicted
1	Mild	≥ 80%
2	Moderate	< 80%
3	Severe	< 50%
4	Very severe	< 30%

Please see www.goldcopd.org for details of classification of severity of airflow limitation in COPD.

Useful background: Performance characteristics of physical examination for COPD

Clinical features	PLR	NLR
o Inspection		
- Maximum laryngeal height <4 cm	3.6	0.7
- Hoover sign	4.2	0.5
o Palpation		
- Subxiphoid cardiac impulse	7.4	NS
o Percussion		
- Absent cardiac dullness left lower sternal border	11.8	NS
- Hyperresonance upper right anterior chest	5.1	NS
o Auscultation		
- Breath sound score		
≤9	10.2	...
10-12	3.6	...
- Early inspiratory crackles	14.6	NS
- Any unforced wheeze	2.8	0.8
o Ancillary tests		
- Forced expiratory time ≥9 seconds	4.1	...

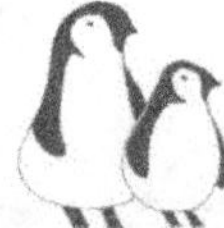

Clinical features	PLR	NLR
o 2 out of the following 3 findings present: - 70-pack-years or more of smoking - Self-reported history of chronic bronchitis or emphysema - Decreased breath sounds	25.7	0.3

Abbreviation: NLR, negative likelihood ratio; NS, not significant; PLR, positive likelihood ratio

Note that some of the clinical features are not shown here, because their PLR is < 2. These include: laryngeal descent >3 cm, diaphragm excursion percussed <2 cm, breathing sound score ≥ 13 and force expiratory time ≤ 9 second.

Adapted from: McGee SR. *Saunders/Elsevier* 2007, Box 30-1, page 361.

SO YOU WANT TO BE A RESPIROLOGIST!

- Give the conditions under which the auscultation of vesicular breath sounds do not signify reduced air flow (e.g., in COPD).
  - Normal thickness of the chest wall
  - Normal pleura (no fluid or air)
  - Normal function of respiratory muscles
  - Reduced/distant breath sounds suggest COPD, as also do vesicular breath sounds. Breath sounds of normal intensity mean that the FEV1 is normal or near normal.
  - Ausculation of the breath sound intensity (BSI) at the bedside (reduced intensity) correlates with FEV1, FEV1/FVC, and distribution of ventilation – a poor person's pulmonary function test – because of airtrapping and destruction of lung parenchyma in COPD
  - In COPD (asthma, chronic bronchitis), the intensity of breath sounds heard at the mouth without the use of a strethoscope increases: with airway obstruction, intensity at mouth increases, over the chest diseases.

Source: Mangione S. *Hanley & Belfus* 2000, page 302.

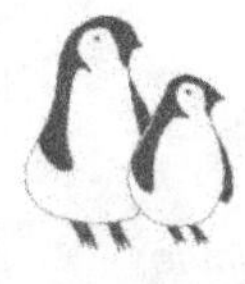

➢ Pulmonary function testing

- Give the spirometry criteria for COPD.
  - FEV_1 < 80% of the predicted value, taken after bronchodilator; plus
  - FEV_1 / FVC < 0.70

- Give the characteristic results of pulmonary function tests in obstructive and restrictive lung diseases.

		Obstructive	Restrictive
Lung volumes	VC	↓	↓
	FRC	↑	↓
	RV	↑	↓
	TLC	↑ or N	↓
Flow rates	FEV 1.0	↓	↓ or N
	FEV 1.0/FVC	↓	↑ or N
	FEF 50% VC	↓	↑ or N
	FEF 25% VC	↓	↑ or N
Diffusion capacity	DCco	↓ or N	↓ or N

Source: Davey P. *Wiley-Blackwell* 2006, page 198.

➢ Differential

Chronic cough, sputum production, and dyspnea are frequent symptoms in the patient with COPD, but these symptoms may be caused by other pulmonary disorders which may masquerade as COPD.

➢ Differential

- Give pulmonary conditions which may **mimic COPD**, and give the clinical features which predict the diagnosis of COPD.
  - Mimics of COPD
    - Upper airway obstruction
    - Emphysema
    - Chronic bronchitis

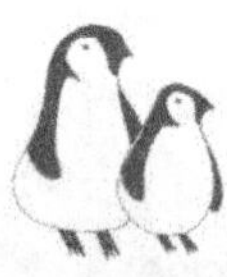

- Bronchiolitis
  - Obliterative (obliterans)
  - Bronchiolitis
- Bronchiectasis
- Cystic fibrosis
- AAT (α-1 antitrypsin)

- Clinical features predictive of COPD
  - > 40-pack-year history of smoking, or
  - History of smoking
  - Wheezing
    - Self-reported
    - On auscultation

Clinical Gem

Note: COPD is <u>not</u> associated with clubbing, unless there is associated disease such as bronchiectasis, TB, or cancer.

➢ Treatment

- Give the therapy of an acute COPD exacerbation.

o Antibiotic	- Mild ▪ TMS (trimethoprim-sulfamethoxazole), or ▪ Tetracycline - Moderate / severe ▪ Fluoroquinolone, or ▪ β-lactam / β-lactamase inhibitor ▪ Macrolide, extended-spectrum ▪ Cephalosporin, second- / third-generation
o Corticosteroids, 2 wk	
o Bronchodilator	- Albuterol - Ipratropium
o Ventilation, non-invasive	- Albuterol plus ipratropium

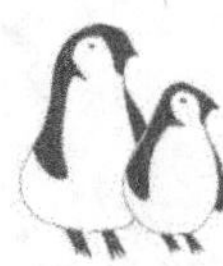

- Maintenance
  - Smoking
    - Stop
  - Vaccination
    - Influenza
    - Pneumococcus
  - FEV1 < 60% of predicted
    - Long-acting inhaled
      - Anti-cholinergics
      - β-agonist
    - Note: do not use both short and long-acting anti-cholinergics together
  - FEV1 < 50% of predicted
    - Pulmonary rehabilitation
  - Continuous O2 therapy
    - Resting or exercise hypoxemia
      - Arterial PO2 < 55 mm Hg, or
      - O2 saturation < 88%
    - Arterial PO2 55-60 mm Hg plus tissue hypoxia
      - Polycythemia
      - PHT (pulmonary hypertension)
      - R-HF (right-sided heart failure)

- Special considerations
  - Consider Low volume reduction surgery, if
    - Upper lobe emphysema, plus
    - Low baseline exercise capacity
    - FEV1 > 20% of predicted
  - AAT (alpha antitrypsin) deficiency
    - Give IV human AAT
  - COPD plus pneumothorax
    - Aspiration, chest tube, pleurodesis, ipsilateral thoracoscopy

- Mechanical ventilation
  - Patients with COPD can be directly weaned from mechanical ventilation to NPPV
  - Patient with primary hypoxemic respiratory failure may be assessed for readiness to be weaned by measuring f/VT (respiratory rate/tidal volume)
  - f/VT > 105 → 80% likelihood of successful weaning off mechanical ventilator
  - NPPV (non-invasive mechanical ventilation)

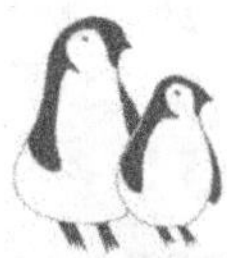

- Low minute ventilation plus permissive hypercapnia to allow sufficient time for exhalation
  - ↓ dynamic expiratory airway collapse, to allow sufficient time for exhalation
  - ↓ airway resistance
  - Avoid
    - Breath stacking
    - Auto-PEEP
- Ventilate to achieve patient's baseline PCO_2

SO YOU WANT TO BE A PULMOLOGIST!

- Give the method to determine if there is auto-PEEP, and how to present breath stacking from occurring.
  - Check EEP (end-expiratory pressure) during end-expiratory pause (no airflow) to determine if auto-PEEP is occurring
  - Prevent breath stacking (delivery of a preset volume before full expiration) by using high inspiratory flow rates

- Give reasons for **chronic ventilator failure** in advanced COPD.
  - ↑ resistance of airways
  - ↓ compliance of chest wall → hyperinflation
  - ↑ ventilation of dead-space

Clinical Pearls

- FEV1 < 50% of predicted
  Use pulmonary rehabilitation of symptomatic COPD
- FEV1 < 60% of predicted
  Use bronchodilators long-term

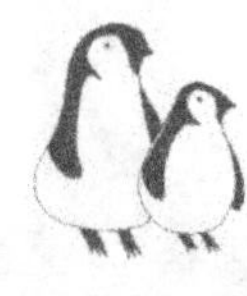

Clinical Gem

- The patient with end-stage COPD has troublesome dyspnea, which may be reduced with morphine extended release, 20 mg per day

Clinical Pearl

- In the patient with COPD who continues to smoke, normal oxygen saturation on pulse oximetry does not exclude arterial hypoxemia, since the carboxyhemoglobin resulting from the smoking would give a false elevation in the reading of the oxygen saturation.
- Assessment of the arterial blood gases would be necessary.

- In the patient with COPD, give the criteria for **LTOT** (long-term O_2 therapy).
    - Arterial $PO_2 \leq 55$ mm Hg, or
    - $O_2 \leq 88\%$ on room air

Special Considerations for COPD

- Longterm
    - Over time, as COPD worsens there is increase in
        - The number of attacks
        - Symptoms

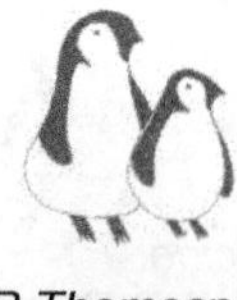

- Pharmaceutical

Monotherapy		Combination Therapy	
FEV1 ≥ 60% of predicted breakthrough symptoms	FEV1 < 60%	FEV1 < 50%	Poor response or adverse effects
- SABA or - SAAch	LABA or LAAch	LABA plus LAAch or ICS plus LABA or LAAch	Add methylxanthine or Phosphodiesterase-4 inhibitor

For details about these medications, please see section on asthma

Abbreviations: ICS, inhaled corticosteroid; LAAch, long-acting anti-cholinergic; LABA, long-acting beta-2 agonist; SAAch, short-acting anti-cholinergic; SABA, short-acting beta-2 agonist

- Corticosteroids (CS)
  - Inhaled
    - Do <u>not</u> use as monotherapy
    - Does <u>not</u> slow the progressive ↓ FEV1
    - ↑ risk of pneumonia associated
  - IV-CS
    - For severe attacks (requiring hospitalization)
  - po-CS
    - Do <u>not</u> use long-term

- Phosphodiesterase-4 inhibitors
  - Oral selective phosphodiesterase-4 inhibitor, roflumilast
  - Mechanism of benefit in COPD not know
  - Not for use in asthma, or emphysema
  - "…. add-on and therapy in patients with severe disease not adequately controlled on other COPD medication" (Source: MKSAP 16 2013, Pulmonary, page 25)
  - Contraindication patients with liver dysfunction

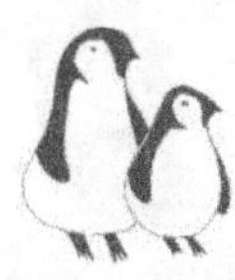

- Care in use
  - Inducers of cytochrome 450
    - Carbamazepine
    - Phenytoin
    - Phenobarbitol
    - Rifampin

Abbreviations: IV, intravenous; po, per os (by mouth)

Treatment advisory

- Do **not** use in COPD
  - Antitussives, since the chronic cough in protective (to clear mucus obstruction)
  - Pulmonary vasodilators
    - Calcium channel blockers
    - NO (nitric oxide)
    - Phosphodiesterase-5 inhibitors
  - Roflumilast in patients with liver dysfunction
  - Morphine in high doses

- Narcotics
  - Morphine
    - Low-doses
      - Useful to ↓ dyspnea
    - High doses
      - Contraindicated (→ hypoventilation)

- Antibiotics
  - Attack
    - Fluoroquinolone, or 3rd – generation cephalosporin plus macrolide
    - Useful when COPD attack caused by
      - Haemophilus influenza
      - Streptococcus pneumonia
      - Moraxella catarrhalis
      - Viral infection (benefit of antibiotics likely against colonization of about bacteria)
      - Severe attack requiring ventilation

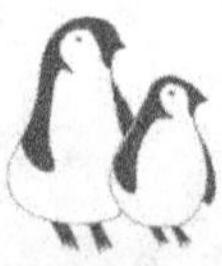

- Prophylaxis
  - No proven benefit to reduce frequency or severity of attacks

- Vaccine
  - Influenza
  - Pneumococcal (7-superior to 23- valent diphtheria-conjugated pneumococcal polysaccharide)

- Non-pharmaceutical
  - Smoking cessation
  - Pulmonary rehabilitation
  - O_2 therapy
  - Mechanical ventilation
  - Lung volume reduction surgery
  - Lung transplantation

- Pulmonary rehabilitation
  - Useful when FEV1 < 50% of predicted
  - Education, nutrition, exercise

- O_2 therapy
  - At home, or in hospital for acute attacks
  - Indications
    - Resting hypoxemia
    - Nighttime/exercise desaturation
    - Cor pulmonale
    - Polycythemia
  - ↑ survival
    - Hospitalization, targets
      - Arterial Po_2 > 60 mm Hg (1.8 kPa), or
      - O_2 saturation > 90%

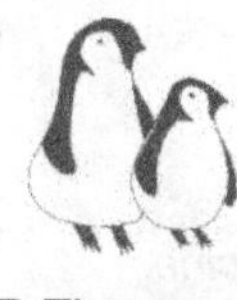

Clinical Alert

- In the hospitalized COPD patient, O_2 therapy is given aggressively to meet target criteria for arterial Po_2 or % O_2 saturation.
- Care is necessary to ensure that there is no CO_2 retention, by performing arterial blood gases 30-60 min after starting O_2 therapy.

➤ Mechanical ventilation, non-invasive

- NPPV (non-invasive positive pressure ventilation)

- Give the indications for NPPV.

  - Indications for NPPV
    - To avoid inturbation in
      - Severe COPD, attack (a "bridge" to avoid invasive (endotracheal inturbation) ventilation
      - Pneumonia/bronchitis
      - Nighttime therapy
      - Rspiratory acidosis (pH < 7.35)
      - Hypercapnea (arterial Pco_2 > 45 mm Hg (6.0 kPa)
      - Respiratory rate > 25 / min

  - Contraindications
    - Please see textbook of pulmonary medicine, or review article such as MKSAP 16 2013, Pulmonary, Table 14, page 27.

➤ Endotracheal Inturbation plus Mechanical Ventilation (CIMV)

- Give 8 medications for EIMV (endotracheal intubation with mechanical ventilation)

  - Severe
    - Respiratory acidosis
      - pH < 7.25
    - Hypercopia
      - Arterial Pco_2 > 60 mm Hg [8.0 kPa]
    - Hyperventilation
      - > 35 / min
    - Hypoxia
    - Respiratory arrest

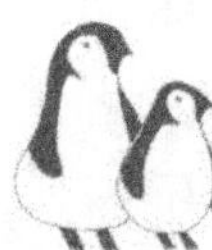

- Complications
  - CNS
    - ↓ LOC (level of consciousness)
  - CVS
    - Hypotension
    - Shock
  - Sepsis
  - Lung
    - Pneumonia
    - Embolism
    - Effusion (very large)
    - Barotrauma

- Lung Volume Reduction Surgery (LVRS)
  - Palliative procedure to remove collapse hyperinflated lung (emphysema → atelectasis)
  - Removing lung develops
    - ↑ elastic recoil
    - ↑ effectiveness of respiratory muscles
    - ↑ expiratory flow rate
    - ↓ air trapping
  - No change in mortality
  - Indications
    - Failure of medical therapy
    - Bilateral upper lobe emphysema on CT scan
    - FEV1 ≤ 45% and > 20% of predicted
    - DLCO > 20% predicted
    - Ambient air arterial Pco_2 ≤ 60 mm Hg (8.0 kPa) plus arterial Po_2 ≥ 45 mm Hg (6.0 kPa)
    - Postbronchodilator TLC (total lung capacity > 150%, plus RLV (residual lung volume) > 100% of predicted

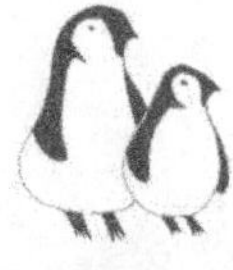

LUNG TRANSPLANTATION

➢ Indications

- Give the criteria for lung transplantation.
    - BODE Index of 7 to 10
    - ≥ 1 of the following
        - Acute hypercapnea Pco_2 > 50 mm Hg (6.7 kPa) with hospitalization
        - PHT (pulmonary hypertension), cor pulmonale, or both despite O_2 therapy
        - FEV1 < 20% of predicted, plus ≥ 1 of the following
            - DLCA < 20% of predicted
            - Distribution of emphysema (upper lobes → homogeneous)
            - Arterial Po_2 < 55 mm Hg (7.3 kPa)

Source: MKSAP 16 2013, Pulmonary, Table 17, page 28.

➢ Outcome

- 1, 3, 5 yr for COPD treated by lung transplantation ~ 80, 60, 40%
- > half develop obliterative bronchiolitis (chronic allograft rejection)

"With self-discipline most anything is possible."
Theodore Roosevelt

BRONCHIECTASIS

- Definition
    - Dilation of bronchii
- Causes/associations
    - Obstruction
    - Infection
    - Fibrosis
    - Rarely congenital

- Perform a focused physical examination for bronchiectasis.
    - Inspection
        - Sputum
            - Purelent
            - Sometimes bloody
        - Evidence of weight loss
        - Kyphoscoliosis
        - Finger clubbing
    - Palpation, percussion, auscultation
        - Bilateral, course crackles on inspiration
        - Signs of
            - Pneumonia
            - Fibrosis
            - Collapse, especially of lower lobes
            - Clubbing
            - Rhonchi
            - Crepitations
            - Effusion
            - Pneumothorax
        - Chest incision
            - One lobe or segment
            - Commonly LLL and lingual

Abbreviation: LLL, left lower lobe

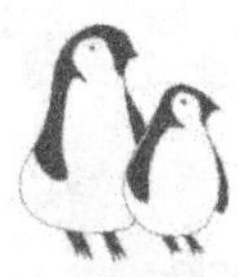

➢ Clinical

- Take a focused history and perform a directed physical examination for bronchiectasis.

- History
  - General
    - Intermittent fever and night sweats
    - Weight loss

  - Lungs
    - Cough with copious purulent sputum
    - Recurrent hemoptysis
    - History of recurrent chest infections
    - History of associated lung disease

- Physical examination
  - Lungs
    - Copious purulent expectoration
    - Collapse
    - Fibrosis
    - Pneumonia
    - Bilateral coarse, late, inspiratory crackles

  - Spine
    - Possible kyphoscoliosis

  - Hands
    - Finger clubbing

  - Spleen
    - Possible splenomegaly (amyloidosis)

Adapted from: Baliga RR. *Saunders/Elsevier* 2007, page 266.

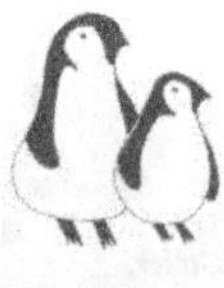

- Perform a focused physical examination for a **pulmonary cavity**.

  - Pathognomonic signs (usually only seen with a large cavity)
    - Percussion (during height of inspiration, with mouth open) – sounds like a cracked pot.
    - Auscultation – when the patient coughs, a hissing sound Is heard

  - Suggestive signs (may be caused by conditions other than cavities).
    - Cavernous breathing
    - Whispered pectoriloquy

SO YOU WANT TO BE RESPIROLOGIST!

- A patient presents with chronic intermittent cough and hemoptysis, but no sputum. There is a past history of pulmonary TB. High resolution CT reveals disease in the upper lobes. Give what this is called.

  - Dry' bronchiectasis, aka bronchiectasis sicca.

- Give the clinical features of diseases associated with bronchiectasis.

	General Clinical Features
Cystic fibrosis	- Due to malfunction of the gene coding for the CF transmembrane conductance regulator (CFTR) protein. Usually diagnosed at a young age - Lung disease often dominates the clinical pictures. - Malabsorption very common; cirrhosis, azoospermia, etc.
Kartegener syndrome	- Due to mutation in gene coding for dynein protein - Ciliary dysmotility, resulting in sinusitis, situs inversus, infertility in men
Young syndrome	- Triad of "bronchiectasis, rhinosinusitis and decreased fertility (obstructive azoospermia)" due to abnormally viscous mucus

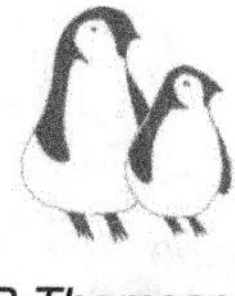

o Immune defects	- IgA deficiency: repeated respiratory tract infections, 25% develop autoimmune conditions (e.g., RA, SLE, celiac disease) IgM deficiency - Recurrent infancy/childhood infections with encapsulated organisms. Later on, autoimmune illnesses and malignancy
o Allergic bronchopulmonary aspergillosis (ABPA)	- Usually complicates long standing asthma, leading to worsening of asthma symptoms - Transient pulmonary infiltrates on chest x-ray - Often with eosinophilia
o Rheumatoid arthritis (RA)	- Bronchiectasis can occur before overt arthritis, though more common with overt RA
o Alpha-1 antitrypsin deficiency	- Chest disease, especially in smokers, at a young age. - Symptomatic liver disease (cirrhosis) occurs at a young age
o Marfan syndrome	- Family history of premature sudden cardiac death, due to aortic dissection - Aortic root enlargement; dissection - Tall, joint hypermobility, lens dislocation

Permission granted: Davey P. *Wiley-Blackwell* 2006, page 195.

➢ Diagnostic imaging

- Give the typical findings on chest X-ray of the patient with bronchiectasis.
  - May be normal, or
  - Fibrosis or collapse (especially at the right heart border)
  - Hilar density
  - Dilated bronchi with “honeycomb” appearance” (dilated bronchi seen as rings with clear centres, within an area of fibrosis)

! Trick Question !

When bronchiectasis is caused by fibrosis from previous TB, in which lobes does the recurrent pneumonia usually occur?

- Upper lobes

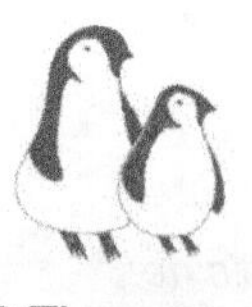

Bode Index

BMI, Obstruction (FEV1), Dyspnea (MMRC), exercise (6-min walk, distance, IM)

Score	BMI	FEV1 % Predicted	MMRC Score	6-Min Walk, M
0	> 21	≥ 65	0-1	≥ 350
1	≤ 21	50-64	2	250-349
2		36-49	3	150-249
3		≤ 35		≤ 149

CYSTIC FIBROSIS (CF)

- Give the bacterial pathogens which most commonly infect the lung of persons with cystic fibrosis (CF), and give the treatment to suppress chronic infection and for acute exacerbations.
    - Common pathogens
        - Pseudomonas aerugenosa
        - Burkholderia cepacia
    - Acute exacerbations
        - Anti-pseudomonal antibiotics
    - Chronic suppression
        - Tobramycin, aerosolized
    - ↑ secretions
        - Hypertonic saline
        - rh DNase (recombinant human DNase)
    - Obstruction
        - Bronchodilators
        - Corticosteroids
    - Immunizations
    - Chest physiotherapy
    - Consider high dose vitamin E therapy
    - Assess and mange nutritional status

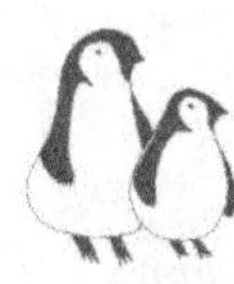

MOUNTAIN SICKNESS (aka HIGH ALTITUDE SICKNESS)

- Types
  - HAPE(high-altitude pulmonary edema)
    - An exaggerated ventilator response to a reduced ambient partial pressure of oxygen, leading to hypocapnia and ventilator instability
    - The ventilator instability leads to cyclic central apneas and hyperapneas associated with repetitive arousals from sleep and paroxysms of dyspnea
  - HACE (high-altitude cerebral edema)
- Treatment
  - Prevention acetazolamide
  - Move to lower altitude (below 1900 [6300 ft])
  - Oxygen/hyperbaric O_2
  - HAPE
    - Furosemide
    - Nifedipine, or
    - Sildenafil
  - HACE
    - Dexamethasone

Adapted from: MKSAP 16 2013, Pulmonary, page 69.

"You are never too old to set another goal or to dream a new dream."

C.S. Lewis

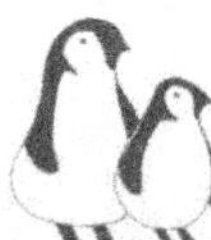

LUNG TUMOURS

- Definition
    - Lesion ≤ 3 cm (diameter) in lung parenchyma
    - Not associated with
        - Other pulmonary lesions
        - Lymphadenopathy
    - Not invading other tissues structures

- Terminology
    - Nodule
        - ≤ 3 cm
        - Focal
        - Single/multiple
        - Surrounding lung, normal
        - Lymphadenopathy, none
    - Mass > 3 cm
    - Likely malignant nodule

- Causes/associations

Of course tobacco smoking (or second-hand smoke) is the major cause of lung cancer.

- Give causes/risk factors of lung cancer, other than tobacco smoking.
    - Airway obstruction (even when seen on PFT [pulmonary function testing])
    - Pulmonary fibrosis
    - Exogenous chemicals
        - Asbestos
        - Hydrocarbons
        - Smoking, or second-hand smoke
        - Metal
            - Arsenic
            - Chromium
            - Nickel
            - Cadmium
    - Family history

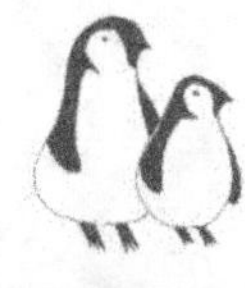

- Radiation
  - To chest
  - To ‘multiple” area
  - Breast cancer
  - Hodgkin lymphoma

➢ Clinical

- Take a focused history for cancer of the lung.
  - Non-specific pulmonary symptoms
  - “B symptoms” (unfortunately, 75% of persons with symptoms from lung cancer already have advanced disease)
  - Mass effect of tumour
  - Symptoms from metastases
    - Lung; lymph nodes
    - Pleura
    - Liver
    - Bones
    - Brain
    - Adrenal glands
  - Symptoms from **paraneoplastic syndromes** (10%)
    - SCLC (small cell lung cancer)
      - CNS
        - Encephalomyelitis
        - Peripheral neuropathy
        - Horner syndrome
          - Infiltration of sympathetic nerves by
          - Tumour in apex of lung
          - Miosis, ptosis, ipsilateral anhidrosis
        - LE-MS (Lambert-Eaton Myasthenic syndrome)
        - Cerebellar ataxia
        - Limbic encephalitis

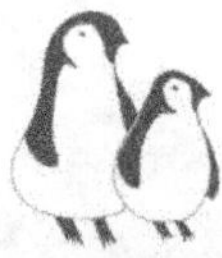

- Paraneoplastic syndromes
  - Result from immune response to tumour or to tumour secretions

- Hypercalcemia	▪ ↑ PTH (parathyroid hormone secreting tumour) ▪ ↑ Ca_s^{2+} usually from bone metastases, rather than ↑ PTH ▪ NSCLC > SCLC
- SIADH secretion	▪ Syndrome of inappropriate ADH [anti-diuretic hormone] secretion ▪ SCLC > NSCLC
- Hypertrophic osteoarthropathy	▪ Clubbing of fingernails ▪ Periostitis ▪ Swollen joints
- Cushing disease	▪ ↑ ACTH (adenocorticorticotropic hormone)

  - Mixed cell types

▪ GI	- Anorexia - Weight loss
▪ MSK	- Clubbing - Hypertrophic osteoarthropathy - Polymyositis - Dermatomyositis
▪ Blood	- Thrombocytosis - Thrombophlebitis - Leukamoid reation
▪ Heart	- Endocarditis, non-bacteria thrombotic

  - Squamous

▪ Endocrine	- Hypercalcemia

- Perform a directed physical examination of the pulmonary system in the patient with suspected mediastinal compression (e.g., carcinoma of the lung).
  - Many patients have no signs
  - General
    - Anorexia
    - Weight loss
    - Cachexia
    - Fever
    - Fatigue

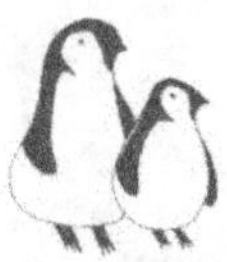

  - Night sweats
  - Cough
  - Dyspnea
  - Purpura (TTP)
  - Hemoptysis
  - Palor (anemia)
  - Voice hoarseness
- CNS
  - Mediastinal nerve compression (sympathetic, left recurrent laryngeal, phrenic nerve)
  - Cortex – dementia
  - Peripheral neuropathy (polyneuropathy, subacute sensory neuropathy)
  - Polymyositis; progressive muscle weakness (Eaton-Lambert syndrome)
  - Retinal blindness (small cell carcinoma)
  - Subacute cerebellar degeneration
  - Polymyositis
  - Cortical degeneration
- Eyes
  - Exophthalmos
  - Horner syndrome
  - Conjunctival redness, venous dilation in the fundi
- Face
  - Plethora
  - Cyanosis
  - Periorbital edema
- Head and neck
  - JVP is raised but not pulsatile
  - Thyroid (large retrosternal goiter) may be supraclavicular lymphadenopathy
  - Metastases
  - Lymphadenopathy
  - SVC obstruction
  - Cushing's syndrome
- Chest
  - Superior vena caval obstruction
    - The face is plethoric and cyanosed with periorbital edema
    - The eyes may show exophthalmos, conjunctival infection, and venous dilatation in the fundi

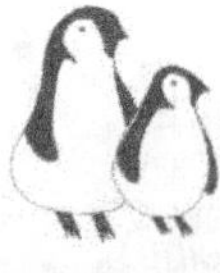

- Lung
  - Consolidation
  - Marks from/for radiation treatment
- Breasts
  - Gynecomastia
- Heart
  - Pericardial tamponade
  - Atrial fibrillation
  - Pericarditis
  - Endocarditis (non-bacterial, thrombotic)
  - Thrombophlebitis migrans
- Metastases
  - Effusion
  - Hemoptyses
  - Lobar collapse or volume loss
  - Pneumonia
  - Fixed inspiratory wheeze
  - Tender ribs (secondary deposits of tumour in the ribs)

- Mediastinal compression
  - Trachea
    - Stridor – respiratory distress
  - Nerve compression
    - Sympathetic nerves – myosis, ptosis, anhydrosis, (Horner's syndrome)
    - Left recurrent laryngeal nerve compression– hoarseness
    - Phrenic nerve-unilateral absent breath sounds; percussion dullness at affected based, with no inspiratory changes (paralysis of diaphragm)
  - Superior Vena Cava (SVC)
    - Pemberton's sign for SVC obstruction – lift arms, wait 1 minute for facial plethora, cyanosis, inspiratory stridor, non-pulsative elevation of JVP
    - Also eyes, face, neck as above

- CNS/ PNS
  - CNS
    - Encephalomyelitis
    - Dementia

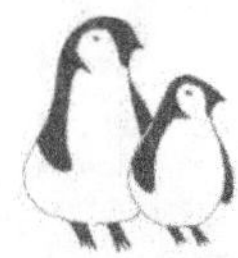

- Cerebellar
  - Degeneration
- Muscle
  - Myopathy (proximal)
  - Neuropathy (sensory)
  - Myoclonus
- PNS
  - Polyneuropathy

- Skin
  - Wasting of small muscles of hands
  - Clubbing
  - Tar staining of fingers
  - Radiation marks
  - Membranous glomerulonephritis
  - Acanthosis nigricans
  - Dermatomyositis (rare)
  - Hypertrophic osteoarthropathy
  - Cigarette stains on fingers
  - Herpes zoster
- Liver metastases
- Bone metastases
- Endocrine
  - Adrenal metastases
  - Hypercalcaemia, due to secretion of parathyroid hormone-like substances, occurs in squamous cell carcinoma
  - Hyponatraemia-antidiuretic hormone is released by small (oat) cell carcinomas
  - Ectopic ACTH syndrome (small cell carcinoma)
  - Carcinoid syndrome (small cell carcinoma)
  - Gynecomastic (gonadotrophins)
  - Hypoglycemia (insulin like peptide from squamous cell carcinoma).
  - Dermatomyositis
  - Acanthosis nigrans
  - Herpes zoster
  - Atrial fibrillation
  - Pericarditis
  - Non-bacterial thrombotic endocarditis
  - Aortic aneurysm (rare)
  - Thyrotoxicosis
  - ↑ADH (↓Na)

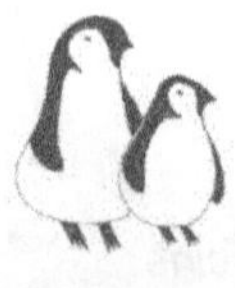

- ↑PTH (↑Ca^{2+})
  - ↑ACTH (hypokalemic alkalosis, Cushing syndrome)
  - ↑Gonadotropins (gynecomastia)
  - ↑ serotonin, carcinoid syndrome
- Hematological features
  - Migrating venous thrombophlebitis
  - Disseminated intravascular coagulaton
  - Anemia
  - TTP
- Kidney
  - Nephritic syndrome (membranous glomerulonephritis)

Abbreviations: CNS, central nervous system; DIC, disseminated intravascular coagulopathy; PNS, peripheral nervous system; SVC, superior vena cava;TTP, thrombotic thrombocytopenic purpura;

Adapted from: Talley NJ, et al. *Maclennan & Petty Pty Limited* 2003, pages 128-129; Davey P. *Wiley-Blackwell* 2006, page 212; Burton JL. *Churchill Livingstone*,1971, pages 33 and 34, Baliga RR. *Saunders/Elsevier* 2007, page 274.

- Give the causes of chest pain in persons with bronchial cancer.
  - Pleurisy
  - Infiltration of intercostals nerves
  - Erosion/infiltration of ribs

- Give a systematic approach to the non-metastatic, non-pulmonary complications of bronchial cancer.

- Endocrine
  - Cushing's syndrome
  - Hypercalcemia
  - SIADH (syndrome of inappropriate ADH)
  - Carcinoid
  - Hypo-/hyperglycemia
  - Thyrotoxicosis
  - Acromegaly
  - Gynecomastia
- Hematology
  - RBC aplasia
  - Polycythemia
  - Hypercoagulable state
  - Hemolytic anemia

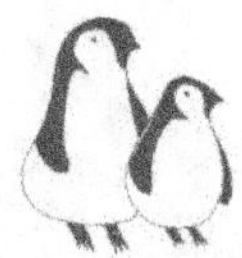

- Neurology (10% of bronchial cancers present with CNS involvement)
  - Benign
    - Dementia
    - Encephalomyelitis
    - Meningitis
  - Cerebellum
  - Cord
    - Corticospinal tract
    - Posterior root ganglion
  - Nerves
    - Neuropathy
    - Mononeuritis multiplex
    - Motor neuron disease
  - Muscle
    - Myopathy
    - Myasthenia
- Skin
  - Dermatomyositis
  - Osteorathropathy
  - Acanthosis migrains
  - Xeroderma
  - Dermatitis herpetiformis
  - Urticaria
  - Exfoliation
  - Tylosis palmars
  - Erythema multiforme
- GI
  - Idiopathic malabsorption
- MSK
  - Dermatomyositis
  - Thrombophlebitis
  - Pulmonary osteoarthropathy

Adapted from: Davies IJT. *Lloyd-Luke (medical books) LTD* 1972, page 135-7.

- Provide a systematic approach to the tumours which are associated with polycythemia.
  - CNS - Cerebellar hemiangiomas
  - Lung - Bronchial carcinoma
  - Liver - Hepatocellular cancer

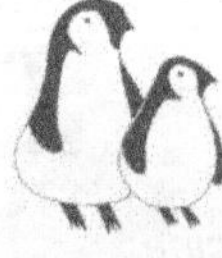

- Kidney
  - Benign tumours
  - Renal cell cancer
- Adrenal
  - Hyperplasia/carcinoma
  - Pheochromocytoma
- GU
  - Ovarian tumours
  - Uterine fibroids

- Give the non-metastatic, extra-pulmonary complications of bronchial carcinoma.

➢ Endocrine
  - Cushing syndrome
  - Hypercalcemia
  - SIADH
  - Hypo-/ hyperglycemia
  - Thyrotoxecosis
  - Acromegaly
  - Gynecomastia

➢ Hematology
  - Red cell aplasia
  - Polycythemia
  - Hemolytic anemia

➢ MSK
  - Dermatomyositis
  - Thrombophlebitis
  - Pulmonary osteoarthropathy

➢ GI
  - Enteropathy

➢ Skin
  - Acanthosis nigricans
  - Dermatitis herpetiformis
  - Urtricaria
  - Erythema multiforme
  - Irritation, exfoliation
  - Tylosis palmaris

➢ Neurological
  - Dementia
  - Encephalomyelitis
  - Cerebellum
  - Spinal cord
  - Corticospinal tract
  - Posterior rectal ganglia
  - Neuropathy
  - Mononeuritis multiplex
  - Myopathy
  - Motor neuron disease
  - Myasthenia gravis

Adapted from: Davies IJT. *Lloyd-Luke (medical books) LTD* 1972, pages 135-7.

SO YOU WANT TO BE A RESPIROLOGIST!

Metastases to the lung are usually seen as a few large deposits.

- Give from what primary tumours are the metastases to the lung usually multiple and small.

  Lung metastasis from primary cancers of

  - Bronchus
  - Stomach

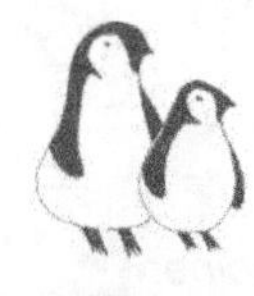

Superior Vena Cava (SVC) **Syndrome**

- Causes of obstruction to SVC
  - Lung cancer
  - Lymphoma
    - Diffuse large B-cell
    - Lymphoblastic

- Diagnosis
  - Chest x-ray
  - Mediastinoscopy plus biopsy
  - CT-guided percutaneous transthoracic needle biopsy

- Treatment
  - Underlying disorder, e.g., chemoradiotherapy
  - Often Rx potency
    - Complete no anti-coagulation
    - Incomplete anti-coagulation

Pulmonary Nodule

- Diagnostic Imaging

- Give the diagnostic imaging features of a solitary pulmonary nodule that suggests **malignancy**.
  - Fuzzy speculated margin
  - No calcification
  - Doubling time on repeat diagnostic imaging (30 to 500 days)

In the context of a solitary pulmonary nodule, for lesions > 1 cm 9diameter), PET scan is positive in 90%.

- Give the conditions which alter the usefulness of PCT scanning to diagnose the cause of solitary pulmonary nodule.
  - Recall that a solitary pulmonary nodule is defined as ≤ 3 cm (diameter)
  - False negative
    - Lesions < 1 cm
  - False positive
    - Any alveolar cell cancer

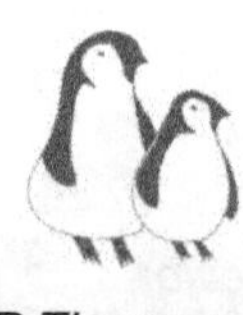

- Give the follow-up recommendations for a pulmonary nodule.

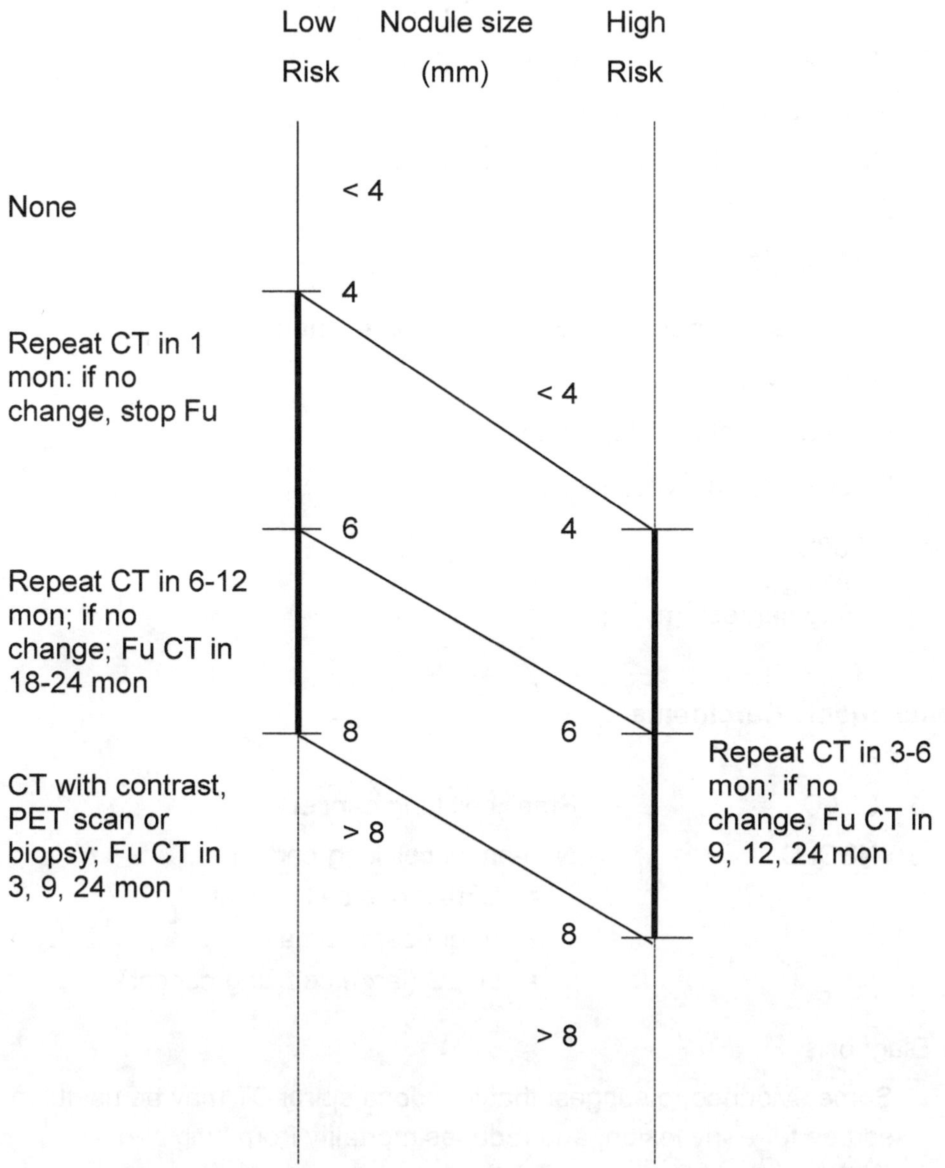

Low Risk | Nodule size (mm) | High Risk

None

< 4

4

Repeat CT in 1 mon: if no change, stop Fu

< 4

6 | 4

Repeat CT in 6-12 mon; if no change; Fu CT in 18-24 mon

8 | 6

Repeat CT in 3-6 mon; if no change, Fu CT in 9, 12, 24 mon

CT with contrast, PET scan or biopsy; Fu CT in 3, 9, 24 mon

> 8

8

> 8

- Give features of a lung nodule which suggests that it may be malignant.
    - History
        - ↑ Age
        - Smoking
        - Other cancer

- Size – < 8 mm, 98% are benign
  – > 20 mm, most are malignant
- Surface – Spiculated
- Associated lymphadenopathy
- Growth of lesion on diagnostic imaging
- Eccentric calcification
- Ground-glass opacity

➢ **Ground-Glass Opacities** (GGO) **Adenocarcinoma**
- Grow slowly
- Limited use of PET for diagnosis
- Biopsy often not diagnostic
- Surgery
  - Wedge resection
  - Segmentectomy

Bronchogenic Carcinoma

➢ Types
- SCLC – Small cell lung cancer
- NSCLC – Non-small cell lung cancer
  - Squamous cell cancer
  - Adenocarcinoma
  - LCLC (large cell lung cancer)

➢ Diagnosis
- Some evidence to suggest that low-dose spiral CT may be useful to screen for early lesion, and reduces mortality from lung cancer (National Lung Screening Trial).
- Diagnosis and staging are done at the same time with
  - CT, or
  - PET CT
  - CT-guided biopsy
  - Bronchoscopy plus biopsy with endoscopic guidance

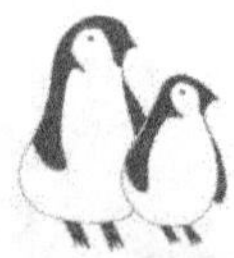

Implication of Findings on CT

- Size
  - See recommendations of Fleischner Society for Thoracic Imaging and diagnosis
  - Doubling time < 50 to 100 days
    - Suspect malignancy
- Calcification
  - Eccentric (off-centre)
    - May be benign or malignant
- Fat
  - Hamartoma
  - Benign
- Satellite nodules
  - Fundus
  - Mycobacteria

  } benign
- PET-CT imaging
  - For detection of malignant is benign nodule
    - Sensitivity, 95%
    - Specificity, 85%
    - Intense activity, think malignant
    - Not useful for
      - < 1 cm nodules
      - GGOs
- Ground-glass opacities (GGOs)
  - Low attenuation (density)
    - Adenomatous hyperplasia
    - Adenocarcinoma
      - In situ (aka bronchioloalveolar carcinoma; adenocarcinoma with lepidic-pattern)
      - Invasive
- Focal
  - Inflammation
  - Fibrosis

- Give the benefit of using **endobronchial ultrasound** to determine resectability of lung cancer.
  - Diagnosis of paratracheal and subcarinal nodes → sensitivity > 90%
  - Negative predictive value → 90%

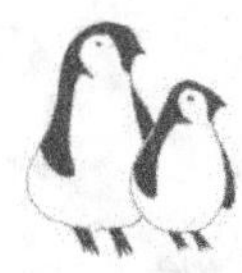

- Screening
  - CT, low dose, spiral
    - High risk smokers > 30-pack-year
    - 20% ↓ mortality from lung cancer mortality
  - Non-calcified nodules
    - > 4 mm
    - < 4 mm, plus
      - Smokers
      - Positive family history
      - Exposure
        - Asbestos
        - Radiation
    - Low-dose spiral CT q 12 mon

  - Malignant pleural effusion represents a distant metastases in the TNM staging system, indicating stage IV disease status. Chemotherapy is for palliation of symptoms, and possibly for prolongation of life

- Staging

  - Used to identify surgically resectable disease
  - Use TNM or VALSE (Veterans Administration Lung Study Group) staging systems
  - "Approximately one in five patients thought to have resectable disease prior to PET-CT will have evidence of mediastinal or distant spread and unnecessary surgery can be avoided" Source: MKSAP 16 2013, Pulmonary, page 60.
- Treatment
  - Surgery, curative-intent
    - Localized disease
      - Stage 1, 1 hemithorax
      - Stage 2, 2 hemithoraxes
    - Low/no cardiovascular risk
    - Acceptable post-operative predicted pulmonary function

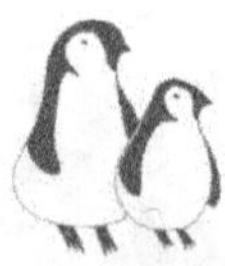

SO YOU WANT TO BE A PULMONOLOGIST!

- In the patient with lung cancer, give the importance of determining FEV_1, and DLCO.
  - As long as there is low or no cardiovascular disease, and the lung cancer is non-metastatic, it is necessary to predict if there will be sufficient pulmonary function after resection of lung tissue (e.g., lobectomy, segment or pneumonectomy)
  - Subtract the amount of lung function that is anticipated to be lost with resection of lung, from the preoperative valve
  - Postoperative predicted FEV_1 and DLCO
    - > 40%
      - Lung resection tolerated
    - < 40%
      - Perform
        - Quantitative perfusion scan, or
        - Exercise assessment of aerobic capacity before rejecting surgical resection

- Lobectomy (promising use of VATS [video-assisted thoracic surgery]), with node dissection
- Post-operative adjuvant chemotherapy for resected stage II
- Non-surgical candidates
  - Radiotherapy
    - Standard
    - Stereotactic
    - Radiofrequency
  - Cryoablation
  - Chemotherapy +/- radiation
    - SCLC
      - Limited stage, chemoradiotherapy
      - Advanced-stage only chemotherapy
- Airway treatment (remove obstructing tumours)
  - Bronchoscopy
    - Laser
    - Cautery
    - Cryotherapy
    - Brachytherapy
    - Stenting

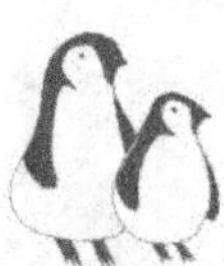

- Give tumours for which adjuvant chemotherapy has been shown to be beneficial.
  - Brain
  - Breast
  - **Lung**
  - GI
    - Esophagus
    - Stomach
    - Pancreas
    - Colon (rectum)

- Give the possible role of genetic testing to direct the treatment of lung cancer.
  - EGFR (epidermal growth factor receptor)
  - ALK (anaplastic lymphoma kinase)

- Give the role of targeted therapy against 3 tumours, using pharmaceutical treatment against VEGF (vascular endothelial growth factors), TKI (tyrosine kinase inhibitors), or EGFR (epidermal growth factor receptor).

Tumour	VEGF-MA	VEGF-TKI	EGFR-MA	EGFR-TKI
Brain	+			
Head and neck			+	
Lung	+		+	+
Breast	+			
Ovary	+			
Liver (HCC)		+		
Pancreas				+
Colon	+		+	
GIST		+		
Renal		+		
CML				+

Abbreviations: CML, chronic myeloid leukemia; EGFR, epidermal growth factor receptor; GIST, gastrointestinal stroma tumour; MA, monoclonal antibody; TKI, tyrosine kinase inhibito

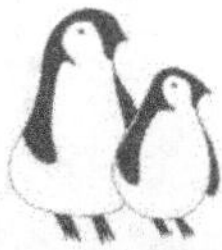

- Give the type or name of targeted therapy against malignant lung tumour.

	Therapies
o VEGF – MA	- Bevacizumab
o EGFR-MA	- Cetuximab, panitumumab
o EGFR-TKI	- Imatinib, gefitnib

SCLC Produce peptide hormones, such as ADH (SIIADH) and ACTH (hypercortisolism).

- Give the neurologic symptoms associated with SCLC.
    - Corticocerebellar degeneration
    - Limbic encephalitis
    - Eaton-Lambert syndrome
    - Peripheral neuropathy

Non-Small Cell Lung Cancer (NSCLC)

Useful background

- More common
- Potentially curable with lung resection
- Histopathology
    - Large cells
        - Subtypes
            - Central squamous
            - Peripheral adenocarcinoma
            - Diffuse brochoalveolar
    - 15% are non-smokers (second-hand smoke), or < 10-pack-year smoking

Stage I	- Only single local primary tumour (peribronchial or hilar)	
IA	- < 3 cm	→ Surgical resection → Chemotherapy

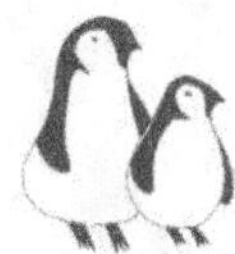

IB - > 3 cm → Surgery plus chemotherapy

Stage II - Primary tumour → Pleura, chest wall, pericarina; or
→ Regional nodes (hilar, peribonchial)

Stage III - Primary tumour → Mediastinal nodes

Stage IV - Primary tumour → Metastasis; or
→ Ipsilateral malignant pleural effusion

➢ Staging

Stage	Tumour	Peribonchial or Hilar Nodes	Mediastinal Nodes	Pleural / Chest Wall Spread near Carina	Metastasis	Ipsilateral Pleural Effusion
Ia	< 3 cm					
B	> 3 cm					
II	+	+	+			
III				+		
IV					+	+

- Stages I to III
    - I - Surgical resection (VATs, video-assisted thoracoscopic surgery)
    - N2 - Ipselateral mediastinal / subcarinal lymph nodes chemotherapy
    - II, III - Post-surgical cisplatin-based chemotherapy (adjuvant chemotherapy)
    - IV - Systemic chemotherapy (2-day platinum-based combination) plus radiation
        - Anti-VEGF bevacizumab or anti-EGF cetuximab
        - EGFR gene mutation in adenocarcinoma
            - Erlotinib (EGFR tyrosine kinase inhibitor)
        - Complications (metastases)
        - Palliation/supportive care
            - Bone, radiation plus bisphosphonate
            - Brain, spinal cord, radiation +/-
            - SVC syndrome, obstructive pneumomitis radiation

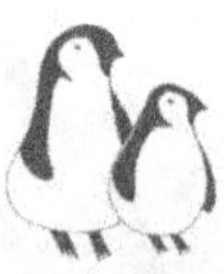

- Treatment
  - Because NSCLC may spreads systemically perform
    - CT chest/abdomen
    - MRI brain contrast-enhanced
    - Bone scan, or PET / CT
  - Mediastinoscopy or bronchoscopic ultrasound with
    - Brushing for cytology
    - Biopsy
  - PFTs (pulmonary function testing)
  - Ventilation scans

Small Cell Lung Cancer (SCLC)

- Useful background
  - Represent 15% of new lung cancers
  - High representation among smokers
  - Usually found proximally in airways
  - Presentation is usually late, with extensive disease
  - Not surgical candidates
  - Early metastases

- Classification
  - Limited disease
    - Hemithorax
  - Extensive disease
    - Hemithorax
      → Ipselateral malignant effusion
      → Metastases
        - Brain
        - Bone
        - Liver

- Treatment
  - Limited disease
    - Chemoradiotherapy (cisplatin or carboplatin, plus etoposide)
    - Initial high response, but > 90% recurrences
    - Prophylactic brain radiation
  - Extensive disease
    - Chemotherapy (cisplatin or carboplatin, plus etoposide or irinotecan)
    - Radiotherapy for palliation of symptoms

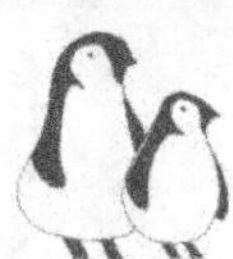

Other Masses in the Mediastinum

- Give differential diagnoses for each of anterior, middle and posterior mediastinal masses.
  - Anterior
    - Thyroid
    - Parathyroid
    - Thymoma
    - Teratoma (aka germ cell tumour)
    - Lymphoma

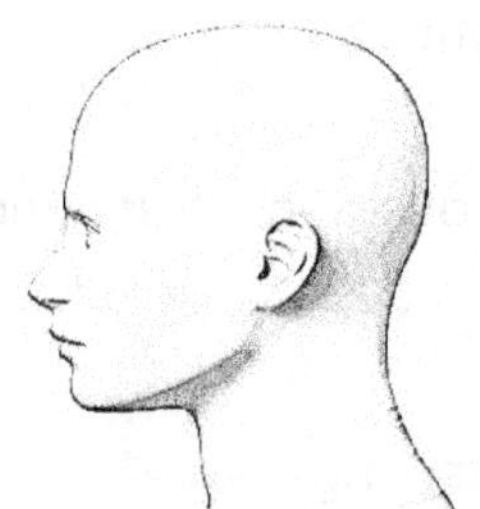

  - Posterior
    - Neural: Neurofibroma, Neurilemmoma
    - Esophagus: Lipoma, Fibroma, Leiomyoma, Carcinoma
  - Middle
    - Lymph nodes
      - Lymphoma
      - Metastasis
      - Granulomatous disease
      - Giant lymph node hyperplasia (Castleman disease)
    - Hiatus (diaphragmatic) hernia
    - Cysts
      - Pericardial
      - Bronchogenic

Carcinoid Tumours

- Low-grade endobronchial malignancy of neuroendocrine cells
- Prognosis
  - Typical — 10-yr survival rate (SR) > 90%
  - Atypical — 5-yr ~ 65%
- Carcinoid syndrome rare (when tumour in lung)

Mesothelioma

- Mesothelial surface of pleura
- Cell types
  - Epithelial
  - Mesotheliomas
  - Mixed
- "Ensheathes" (grows to surround) lung
- 75% of persons with mesothelioma have asbestos exposure
- Treatment
  - Extrapleural pneumonectomy (remove lung plus pleura)
  - Chemotherapy
  - Pleurodesis

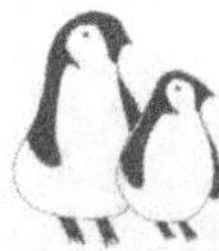

Metastatic disease

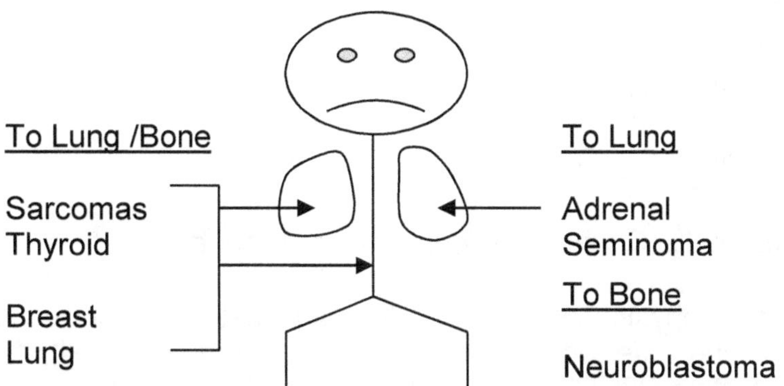

Adapted from: Burton JL. *Churchill Livingstone*, 1971, page 34.

- Causes of mediastinal tumours
  - Lymphadenopathy
    - Reticulosis
    - Sarcoidosis
    - Infective (especially TB)
    - Metastasis
  - Heart
    - Aneurysm
    - Tumour
    - Pericardial cysts
  - Aorta
    - Unfolding
    - Aneurysm
    - Coarctation
  - Esophagus
    - Hiatus hernia
    - Corkscrew
    - Achalasia
    - Enterogenous cyst
    - Neoplasm
  - Thyroid
    - Retrosternal goiter
  - Cysts
    - Dermoid
    - Teratoma
    - Hydatid cysts
    - Bronchial cysts

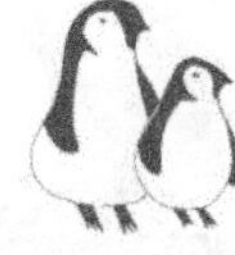

- Tumours
  - Thymoma
- Diaphragm
  - Diaphragmatic hernia
  - Lung herniation
  - Mesothelioma
  - Lipoma

Adapted from: Burton JL. *Churchill Livingstone* 1971, page 34.

- Perform a directed physical examination for Pancoast (superior pulmonary sulcus tumour) syndrome (often from cancer [often non-small cell] of the apex of the lung, infiltrating C8, T1, 2; may also occur with lymphoma, or by spread of lymph node metastases in breast or lung cancer).
  - Shoulder pain radiating in the ulnar distribution in the arm
  - Numbness of digits #4,5
  - Weakness of hand muscles innervated by ulnar nerve
  - Radiologic destruction of ribs #1,2
  - Horner's syndrome

Adapted from: Davey P. *Wiley-Blackwell* 2006, page 212.

AV Malformation

A patient presents with hemolysis and pulmonary nodules are found on chest X-ray.

- Perform a focused physical examination for possible pulmonary AVMs (arteriovenous malformation)
  - CNS
    - CVA
    - Brain abscess
  - Face
    - Mucocutaneous tenangiectasias
    - Cyanosis
    - Polycythemia
  - Hands
    - Clubbing
    - Polycythemia
  - Lung
    - Hypoxemia
- Give the treatment for symptomatic or large (> 2 cm) pulmonary AVMs.
  - Embolotherapy
  - Surgery

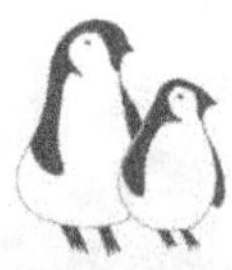

PULMONARY VASCULAR DISEASE

Pulmonary hypertension and Cor pulmonale

- Definition
  - Pulmonary artery pressure > 40 mm Hg
  - "……..a general term for disorders that directly narrow the lumen of small pulmonary arteries and arterioles, raising pulmonary vascular resistance and pulmonary artery pressure"
    Source: BB 2013, page 299.
  - Pulmonary hypertension as an ↑ PAP (pulmonary artery pressure) ≥ 25 mm Hg when the patient is at rest.

- Types
  - The importance of the classification of pulmonary hypertension is that the idiopathic form of pulmonary arterial hypertension (PAH) is treated differently than other forms in which there may be a treatable condition leading to the pulmonary hypertension.

- Classify pulmonary hypertension and give causes/associations.
  - Pulmonary arterial hypertension
    - Resting mean PAP ≥ 25 mm Hg
    - PCWP ≤ 15 mm Hg (normal)
    - ↑ pulmonary vascular resistance
      - Idiopathic (aka primary pulmonary hypertension)
      - Inherited
        - Congenital heart disease
        - Mutations in BMPR2
      - Inflammatory
        - Connective tissue diseases
      - Infection
        - HIV
        - Schistosomiasis
      - Iatrogenic
      - Hematology
        - Chronic hemolytic
      - GI
        - Cirrhosis
        - Portal hypertension

o Left-sided heart disease	- mPAP > 25 mm Hg - PCWP > 15 mm Hg - Left-sided heart dysfunction Systolic or diastolic dysfunction Valvular disease
o Lung disease +/- hypoxia	- mPAP > 25 mm Hg - Underlying lung disease - COPD - Mixed obstruction and restriction - Interstitial lung disease - ↓ alveolar ventilation disorders - Abnormal breathing in sleep

- o Pulmonary veno-occlusive disease disease +/- capillary hemangiomatosis
- o Chronic thromboembolic disease
- o Miscellaneous
  - Long list of associations, e.g.,

▪ Endocrine	- Thyroid disease
▪ Hematology	- Myeloproliferative disorders - Sickle cell disease
▪ Kidney	- CFR on dialysis
▪ Lung	- Langerhans cell histiocytosis - Vasculitis
▪ Infiltration	- Tumour obstruction
▪ Idiopathic	- Fibrosing mediastinitis
▪ Inflammation	- Sarcoidosis

Abbreviations: COPD, chronic obstructive pulmonary disease; CRF, chronic renal failure; mPAP, mean pulmonary arterial pressure; PCWP, pulmonary capillary wedge pressure

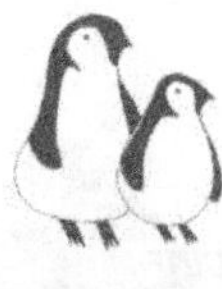

➢ Causes

- Give causes of pulmonary hypertension (PHT) in which screening should be undertaken.

  - Family – First degree relative with familial PHT
  - Heart – Congenital heart disease
    - S → P (systemic [L] to pulmonary [R] shunt
  - Lung – Scleroderma (limited cutaneous, not diffuse cutaneous SSC)
    – CTEPH (chronic thromboembolic pulmonary hypertension)
  - Liver – Cirrhosis (portal hypertension), with symptoms or signs suggestive of PH

➢ Pathophysiology

Persons with increased body mass index (BMI) or drug abuse may be at increased risk for the development of PH (pulmonary hypertension).

- Give the mechanism of development of pulmonary hypertension after pulmonary embolization.

  - After an acute PE (pulmonary embolus), thromboemboli may remain in the pulmonary arteries
  - These thromboemboli may become remodeled, causing scars which ↑ pulmonary vascular resistance → PH
  - ↑ mPaP; PCWP, normal; ↑ PVR (pulmonary vascular vascular resistance)
  - ↓ expression of vasodilators
    - Prostacyclin
    - NO (nitric oxide)
  - ↑ expression of vasoconstrictors
    - Endothelin
  - ↑ expression of growth factors (GF)
    - Endothelial-derived
    - Platelet-derived

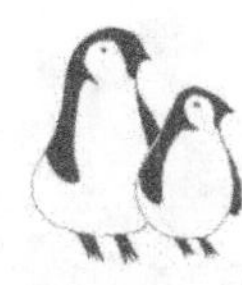

➢ Clinical

- Perform a focused physical examination for pulmonary hypertension.
  - Inspection
  - Palpation
    - RV heave
  - Auscultation
    - Heart sounds
      - ↑ S2, pulmonary component (↑ P2)
      - S3 or S4 RV gallop
    - Murmur
      - TR (tricuspid regurgitation)
      - PI (pulmonary insufficiency)
  - Signs of underlying disorder, e.g.,
    - SLE (systemic lupus erythematosus)
    - SSC (systemic sclerosis)

➢ Diagnosis

o Cardiac	- Ultrasound - Catheterization, right side
o Lung	- Chest X-ray - CTA - V / Q scan - PFT with DLCO - 6-min walk test - Studies for associated conditions

Abbreviations: CTA, CT angiography; PFT, pulmonary function test; DLCO, diffusion capacity ith carbon monoxide

- Give tests used to investigate possible PHT (pulmonary hypertension).
  - Chest X-ray (neither sensitive nor specific for PHT)
  - Echocardiogram, +/- bubble contrast
  - TEE (transesophageal echocardiogram)
  - Catheterization, right heart ± vasoreactivity test
  - Vasoreactivity test (↓ pulmonary artery pressure)
  - PFTs (pulmonary function tests)
  - Polysomnography (if clinical suspicion of OSA [obstructive sleep apnea])

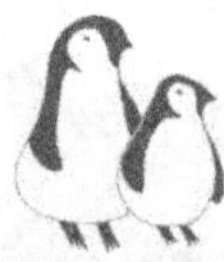

Cor Pulmonale

- Definition: Cor pulmonale is right ventricular enlargement due to the increase in afterload that occurs in diseases of the lung, chest wall or pulmonary circulation.

- Causes
  - Obstructive lung disease
    - COPD
    - Chronic asthma
  - OSA (obstructive sleep apnea)
  - Vasoconstriction secondary to hypoxia
    - High altitude
    - Chronic bronchitis
  - Restrictive lung disease
    - Intrinsic
      - interstitial fibrosis
      - lung resection
    - Extrinsic
      - Obesity
      - muscle weakness
      - kyphoscoliosis
      - high altitude
  - Vascular disorders
    - Pulmonary emboli
    - Vasculitis (small pulmonary arteries)
    - ARDS
    - Primary pulmonary hypertension
  - Heart
    - L-CHF
    - Pulmonary venous hypertension (MS, atrial myxoma, cortriatriatum)
    - Congenital heart disease, L-R shunt (ASD, VSD, PPA)
  - Spine
    - Kyphoscoliosis
    - Ideopathic (primary)

Abbreviations: BMI, body mass index; JVP, jugular venous pressure; L-CHF, Left-sided congestive heart failure; R-CHF, Right-sided congestive heart failure; CO, Cardiac output; PA, pulmonary artery; SPAP, systolic pulmonary artery pressure; COPD, Chronic obstructive pulmonary disease; RR, Respiratory rate; TR, tricuspid regurgitation PA

Adapted from: Baliga RR. *Saunders/Elsevier* 2007, pages 269 and 270.

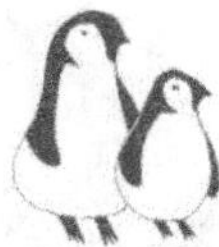

➢ Clinical

- Perform a focused physical examination for cor pulmonale.

➢ General
- Dyspnea at rest (↑ RR)
- Cyanosis
- Fatigue
- ↑ BMI (obesity)
- Kyphoscoliosis

➢ Neck
- ↑ JVP
- 'a' & 'v' waves on JVP
- ↑ v waves with TR
- Hoarseness (PA compression of L. recurrent laryngeal nerve)

➢ Chest
- Chest wall
  - Barrel-shaped
  - L. parasternal heave
- Lung
  - COPD
  - Bilateral wheeze
  - Chronic asthma
  - Fibrosis
  - Resection
- Heart
  - ↓ pulse volume (↓CO)
  - ↑ JVP both 'a' and 'v' waves are seen, 'v' waves being prominent if there is associated tricuspid regurgitation
  - RV heave, gallop
  - Palpable P_2, loud P_2 (forceful valve closure due to ↑ SPAP)
  - Systolic ejection click (PA dilated)
  - S_4
  - Pulmonary ejection murmur (PA dilation with turbulent flow)
  - Pulmonary regurgitation (PA dilation)
  - ↑ P2
  - Ejection click
  - TR (pansystolic murmur)
  - Graham Steell murmur (early diastolic murmur in pulmonary area)

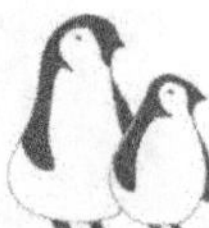

- Abdomen
  - Hepatomegaly
  - RUQ
    - Tender
    - Murmur
    - Thrill (TR)
- Limbs
  - Edema
  - Cold
  - Tar stained fingers

Deep Vein Thrombosis

Useful background: EBM-carotid artery stenosis and deep vein thrombosis

- Gold standard for diagnosing DVT is venography, however it is invasive. Compression ultrasonography is highly sensitive, specific for detecting proximal DVTs and is less invasive.
- A simplified clinical model was generated to stratify individuals into pre test categories of low (score <0), moderate (score 1-2), or high risk (score >3) for DVT. Combining this with compression ultrasonography determined positive likelihood ratios.
- In patients with TIA, a carotid bruit indicated the presence of a >50% stenosis of the carotid artery (confirmed by carotid angiography) with 29% sensitivity and 88% specificity.

Source: Likelihood of Pulmonary embolism according to scan category and clinical probability in PIOPED study *JAMA* 1990; 263:2753.

Note that a number of historical features are not given points for the calculation of the wells score for DVT; these include:

- Stasis – immobilization, right-sided heart failure, obstruction, shock
- Hypercoagulability, estrogen use, pregnancy, neoplasms, tissue trauma, nephritic syndrome, deficiency of antithrombin III, protein C or S
- Endothelial damage – venulitis, trauma
- Symptoms suggesting pulmonary emboli (dyspnea, pleuritic chest pain, and hemoptysis)

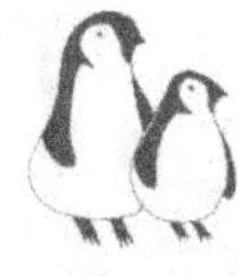

Pretest probability	Sensitivity (%)	Specificity (%)	Positive LR	Probability of DVT (%)
o Low (0)	2-21	36-77	0.2	5
o Moderate (1-2)	13-39	…	NS	17
o High (≥ 3)	38-87	71-96	5.2	53

Abbreviation: NS, not significant

Adapted from: Hauser SC, et al. *Mayo clinic Gastroenterology and Hepatology Board Review. 3rd Review*, page 617; Simel, DL, et al. *JAMA* 2009, Table 18-14, page 246.

Useful background: Likelihood ratios for pulmonary embolus for the combination of clinical probability estimate with the D- dimer result

Clinical Probability	D-dimer	
o Any probability	Abnormal	1.7
o Low (<15%) to moderate (15%-35%)	Normal	0

CI, confidence interval; LR, likelihood ratio

Source: Simel, DL, et al. *JAMA* 2009, Table 43-3, page 575

- Take a directed history and perform a focused physical examination to determine the possible presence of a deep vein thrombosis (DVT).

Wells Scoring Scheme for pretest probability of **DVT**

Clinical Feature	Points
➢ Risk factors	
o Active cancer	1
o Paralysis, paresis or recent plaster immobilization of the lower extremities	1
o Recently bedridden > 3 days or major surgery within 4 weeks	1

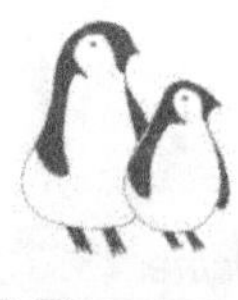

Clinical Feature	Points
➢ Signs	
o Localized tenderness along the distribution of the deep venous system	1
o Entire leg swollen	1
o Asymmetric calf swelling (>3 cm difference, 10 cm below tibial tuberosity)	1
o Asymmetric pitting edema	1
o Collateral superficial veins (nonvaricose)	1
➢ Alternative diagnosis	
o Alternative diagnosis as likely or more likely than deep venous thrombosis	-2
	Total

*Interpretation of score: High probability if 3 points or more, moderate probability if 1 or 2 points and low probability if 0 points or less.

Source: Hauser SC, et al. *Mayo Clinic Gastroenterology and Hepatology Board Review. 3rd Review,* page 617.

- Give the **Simplified** Wells Scoring System for pretest probability of DVT.

Findings in the simplified Wells Scoring system	Score
o Clinical signs/symptoms of DVT of the leg (minimum of leg swelling and pain with palpation of the deep veins)	3.0
o No alternate diagnosis that is as likely as or more likely than a pulmonary embolus	3.0
o Heart rate > 100/min	1.5
o Immobilization or surgery in the last 4 weeks	1.5
o History of DVT or PE	1.5
o Hemoptysis	1.0
o Cancer actively treated in the past 6 months	1.0

Abbreviations: DVT, Deep Vein thrombosis; PE, pulmonary embolism
Category scores determined by the sum of the individual scores: low, <2; moderate, 2-6; high, >6.

Source: Simel DL, et al. *JAMA* 2009 Chapter 43, Table 43-12, page 575.

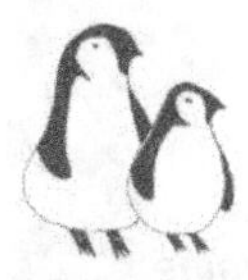

- Give the differential diagnosis of an acute painful calf.
    - DVT
    - Ruptured Baker cyst (herniation of fluid filled synovium of posterior knee)
    - Ruptured gastrognemius muscle

Useful background: Probability of deep vein thrombosis after first determining the clinical probability and then obtaining the D dimer result

		Probability of DVT after applying D dimer Result to the clinical probability estimate, %		
Clinical probability estimates[a]		High probability (~50%)	Moderate Probability (~20%)	Low probability (~5%)
o High sensitivity D-dimer	Positive	63	25	11
	Negative	8.6	1	0.5
o Moderate sensitivity D-dimer	Positive	67	34	17
	Negative	19	4.4	0.9

Abbreviation: DVT, Deep vein thrombosis

Values in the Table use the exact summary pretest probability estimates, but a clinician might simplify by remembering that a high probability is about 50%, moderate probability 20% and low probability 5%.

Source: Simel DL, et al. *JAMA* 2009, Table 18-15, page 246.

SO YOU WANT TO BE A PEDIATRIC RESPIROLOGIST!

- In the context of deep vein thrombosis (DVT), what is Virchow triad?
    - Damage to the vessel wall
        - Trauma
        - Hypoxic blood
        - Drugs
        - Infection
        - Cholesterol
    - ↓ blood flow
    - ↑ blood coagulability

Source: Baliga RR. *Saunders/Elsevier* 2007, pages 100 and 101.

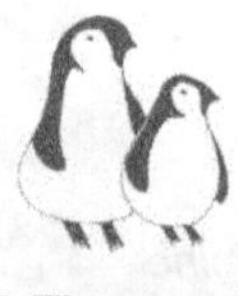

ACUTE PULMONARY THOMBOEMBOLISM

- Risk factors
  - Commonest cause
    - DVT (deep vein thrombosis)
    - ~ 20% of DVT → PE (pulmonary embolus)
  - ↑ coagulability
    - Inherited
    - Acquired
  - Stasis
  - Endothelial damage

For an outline of the many causes of hypercoagulability, venous stasis and endothelial damage, refer to any textbook of internal medicine, a recent article such as UpToDate or MKSAP 16 2013, Pulmonary, Figure 13, page 47; or N Engl J Med 2008, 358: 1037-1052.

- Pathophysiology
  - Thrombus obstruction of portions of pulmonary vasculature
  - ↑ pressure in PA (pulmonary artery) and RV (right ventricle)
  - ↓ CO (cardiac output)
  - Mismatching of ventilation (V) with perfusion (Q)
    - V/Q mismatch
  - ↓ gas exchange

- Clinical assessment
  - The symptoms and signs of PE (pulmonary embolus) are non-specific
  - Take a history for hypercoagulability, venous stasis, endothelial damage
  - Perform a focused physical examination for
    - ↑RR, ↑ HR, ↑ P2, ↑ JVP;
    - Signs of DVT, pulmonary crackles, and hemodynamic status
  - Use clinical risk prediction (Walls, or Revised Geneva) scores of pretest probability of PE

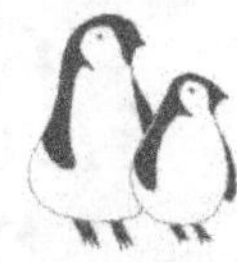

- The pretest probability of PE (low, intermediate, high) will direct which investigation to perform next, e.g.,

  measure
  - Low probability of PE in a hemodynamically stable patient ⟶ if negative, diagnosis, unlikely to be PE D-dimer
  - High probability or hemodynamically unstable patient ⟶ CTA (CT angiography)

SO YOU WANT TO BE A PULMONOLOGIST!

- In the context of the patient with a possible PE (pulmonary emboli), give the meaning of the Hampton hump and the Westermark sign on chest X-ray.

  - Hampton hump
    - Triangular opacity
    - Rounded apex
    - Pleura-based
  - Westermark sign
    - Hyperlucent area

- Give the **Wells Prediction Score** for Pretest Probability of **PE.**

Clinical variable	Points
DVT suspected from symptoms and signs	3.0
PE is likely diagnosis	3.0
HR > 100 bpm	1.5
Immobilization or surgery within 4 wk	1.5
DVT or PE previously	1.5
Hemoptysis	1.0
Cancer	1.0
Total Wells score	12.5

Modified from MKSAP 16 2013, Pulmonary, Table 34, page 48; copyright 2000, International Society on Thrombosis and Haemostasis.

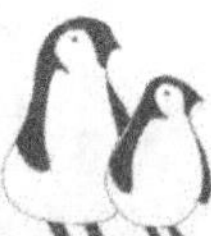

- Interpretation of Wells Score

Pretest probability of PE	Total Well's Score
- Low	< 2.0
- Intermediate (moderate)	≤ 4 PE unlikely → measure D-dimer 2.0-6.0 > 4 PE likely → perform CTA
- High	> 6.0

Abbreviations: bpm, beats per minute; CTA, CT angiogram; DVT, deep vein thrombosis; HR, heart rate; PE, pulmonary embolus

Source: Likelihood of Pulmonary embolism according to scan category and clinical probability in PIOPED study *JAMA* 1990; 263:2753.

Simplified Clinical Model	Score
o Active cancer (treatment ongoing or within previous 6 months or palliative	1
o Paralysis, paresis, or recent plantar immobilization of lower extremity	1
o Recently bedridden for >3 days or major surgery within 4 weeks	1
o Localized tenderness along the distribution of the deep venous system	1
o Entire leg swelling	1
o Calf swelling >3cm, compared to other calf (10cm below tibial tuberosity)	1
o Pitting edema (greater in symptomatic leg)	1
o Collateral superficial veins (non-varicose)	1
o Alternate diagnosis as likely or greater than DVT	-2
	Total

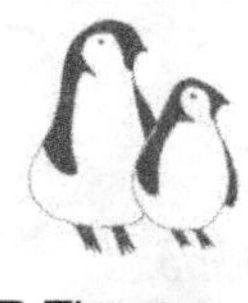

➢ **Revised Geneva Scoring System** for Pretest Probability of Pulmonary Embolism

Clinical Variable	Points
o HR ≥ 95 bpm	5
o Lower limb pain on deep palpitation plus unilateral edema	4
o Unilateral lower limb pain	3
o Previous DVT or PE	3
o HR 75-94 bpm	3
o Hemoptysis	2
o Surgery (under general anesthesia) or fracture lower limbs within 1 mon	2
o Active cancer (solid or hematologic, currently active considered cured < 1 yr	2
o Age > 65 yr	1
Total revised Geneva score	25

Modified from MKSAP 16 2013, Pulmonary, Table 35, page 48; copyright 2006, American College of Physicians.

- o Interpretation of revised Geneva Score

Pretest Probability of PE	Total Geneva Score
- Low	0-3
- Intermediate	4-10
- High	≥ 11

➢ Diagnosis

- o Clinical
  - Use validated Wells or revised Geneva Score to establish pretest probability, and from here proceed with choice of investigations
    - ▪ Biochemistry blood tests
    - ▪ ECG (electrocardiography)
    - ▪ Chest X-ray
    - ▪ CTA (CT angiography)
    - ▪ V/Q lung scan
    - ▪ Compression ultrasound of lower legs
    - ▪ Pulmonary angiography
  - o If PE found, then for predisposing factors e.g., cancer, coagulation abnormalities

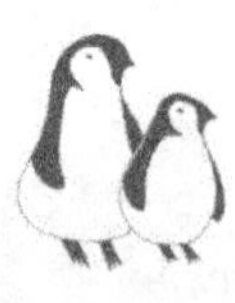

- Biochemical Blood Tests
  - D-dimer
    - A negative test
      - In a patient with low clinical pretest probability of PE, in a patient who is hemodynamically stable basically excludes PE as a diagnosis.
      - In a patient with intermediate or high probability of PE on Wells or Revised Geneva score, the D-dimer is of limited use regardless of a positive or negative result.
  - Markers of cardiac dysfunction
    - Do not help to decide choice of heparin or thrombolytic therapy
    - When positive in a patient with PE, markers of cardiac dysfunction suggest a poorer prognosis, and guide possible use of thrombolysis
    - These tests include
      - Blood tests
        - ↑ BNP (B-type naturetic peptide)
        - ↑ troponin
        - ↓ Na^+_s
      - Cardiac ultrasound showing right heart strain

- Chest X-ray
  - Useful to exclude other diagnosis, or extent of pre-existing lung disease
  - Most findings arising from possible PE are non-specific
    - Atelectasis
    - Raised hemidiaphragm
    - Pleural effusion
      - Unilateral
      - < 1/3 of hemithorax
  - Two chest X-ray findings of PE are not sensitive but are more specific
    - Westermark sign
      - Focal hyperlucent area distal to PE
    - Hampton
      - Cone-shaped density at the periphery of the lung, with the base of the cone apposed to the wall of the chest

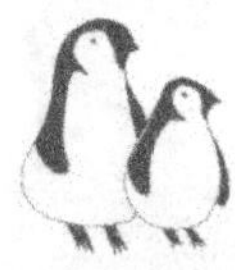

- Echocardiography

- GIVE THE ECG CHANGES IN PULMONARY EMBOLISM.
    - Sinus tachycardia
    - Tall R wave in lead VI
    - S1, S2, S3 syndrome (S waves in limb leads I, II and III)
    - S1, Q3, T3 syndrome (S in limb lead 1 and Q wave and inverted T wave in limb lead III)

Source: Baliga RR. *Saunders/Elsevier* 2007, page 257.

Useful background: ventilation – perfusion scan

	Ventilation	Perfusion
o PE	N	↓
o Pneumonia	↓	↓

Abbreviation: PE, pulmonary embolus; N, normal

If patient is hemodynamically unstable and cannot have CTA or V/Q scan, echocardiography may provide evidence of right heart strain.

SO YOU WANT TO BE AN ECHOCARDIOGRAHER!

- Give the signs on echocardiogram which indicate right heart strain, and support (but so not establish) the diagnosis of PE.
    - The signs on echocardiography which support the diagnosis of PE include
        - ↑ PASP (pulmonary artery systolic pressure)
        - ↑ RV (dilation of right ventricle)
        - ↓ LV (↓ size of left ventricle)

➢ Treatment

- Hemodynamic stability
  - Immediate anti-coagulation with heparin plus warfarin, weaning heparin by day 5 when INR therapeutic at between 2.0 to 3.0 for 2 consecutive days, and adjusting the dose of heparin based on aPTT (activated partial thromboplastin time), or when using LMWH, monitor plasma levels of Xa
  - Observe usual caution re contraindications to anti-coagulation
  - Duration of anti-coagulation (A/C)
    - Known risk factors are correctable
      - A/C for 3 mon
    - Risk factors
      - Unknown
      - Cancer
      - Proximal DVT
      - ↑ D-dimer after stopping A/C for 3-4 wks
      - A/C indefinitely
  - In CRF (Chronic renal failure)
    - Precaution using LMWH, fondaparinax, rivaroxaban (Xa inhibitor)
  - In HIT (heparin-induced thrombocytopenia)
    - Use hirudin, bivalirubin, argatroban
  - High risk patient or high risk of recurrent emboli when A/C unsuccessful or contraindicated
    - IVC (inferior vena cava) filters

- Hemodynamic instability
  - Consider IV thrombolytic therapy
    - Shock
    - Cardiac arrest
    - Severe PE (pulmonary embolus with hypotension)
    - Note: IV thrombolytic therapy for PE does not ↓ mortality rate
  - Strong contraindications to anti-coagulation
    - IVC filter
    - Embolectomy

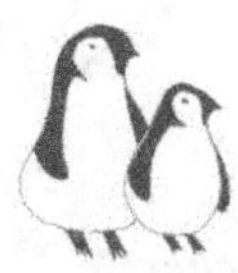

SO YOU WANT TO BE A RESPIROLOGIST!

- In the context of a pleural effusion seen on a lateral chest X-ray, give the meaning of the "Ellis S-shaped line".
    - The Ellis S-shaped line is an S-shaped line seen in the axilla of a patient with an effusion which is encapsulated or associated with air.

- For the following clinical situation, indicate the appropriate VTE (venothromboembolic) prophylaxis.

Surgical procedure	UFH	LMWH	Fondaparinux	Warfarin IPC
o General high risk	√	√	√	
o Cancer		√		+
o Orthopedic - Arthroplasty hip / knee - Fracture hip		√	√	√
o Spinal cord		√	√	√
o Trauma (serious)		√	√	√
o Hospitalized medical patients	√	√		
o Active cancer		√		
o ↓ renal function (GFR < 30 mL /min per 1.73 m^2)		Adjust dose	Contraindicated	

- HIT
    - Recombinant hirudin (lepirudin), or argatroban

Abbreviations: HIT, heparin-induced thrombocytopenia; IPC, intermittent pneumatic compression; LMWH, low molecular weight heparin; UFH, unfractionated heparin

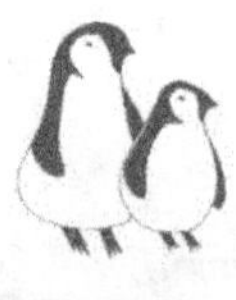

- Give the duration of anti-coagulation after a pulmonary embolus (PE).

Episode	Risk factors	Duration
○ First episode	– Risk factors ▪ Present ▪ Correct	As long as risk factors present 3-6 mon
	– No risk factors (idiopathic)	Life-long
○ Recurrent	– Idiopathic	Life-long
○ Anti-phospholipid antibody syndrome		Life-long

Air travel

- Cabin pressurization reduces inspired O_2 tension from a normal of ~ 160 to 120 mm Hg
- In persons with PH (pulmonary hypertension) or COPD, this causes ↓ arterial oxygenation
- Hypoxia → ↑ PAP (pulmonary artery pressure) results in leaky vasculature and pulmonary edema
- Oxyhemoglobin saturation < 92% → need for in-flight supplemental O_2

ACUTE RESPIRATORY DISTRESS SYNDROME (ARDS)

➢ Definition: "….a syndrome of hypoxemic respiratory failure due to alveolar damage and the leakage of fluid across the alveolar-capillary barrier (non-cardiogenic pulmonary edema)" (BB 2013, page 292)

- "Berlin criteria"
  - Acute onset within 1 week of an apparent clinical insult, or
  - Development and progression of respiratory symptoms
  - Bilateral opacities on chest imaging (chest X-ray or CT imaging) not explained by other pulmonary pathology

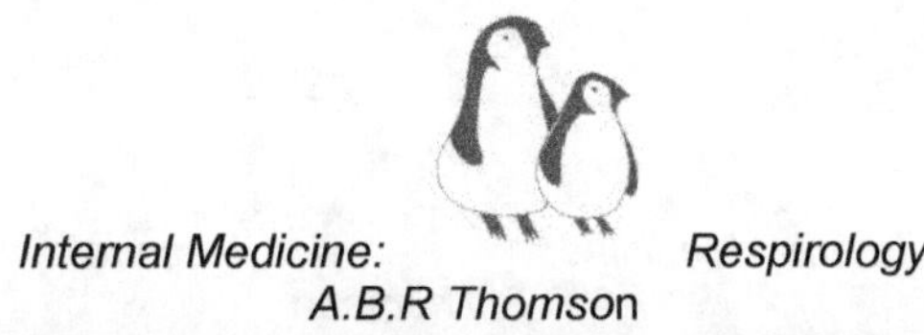

- Pathophysiology
  - Non-cardiogenic pulmonary edema
  - Hypoxemic respiratory failure

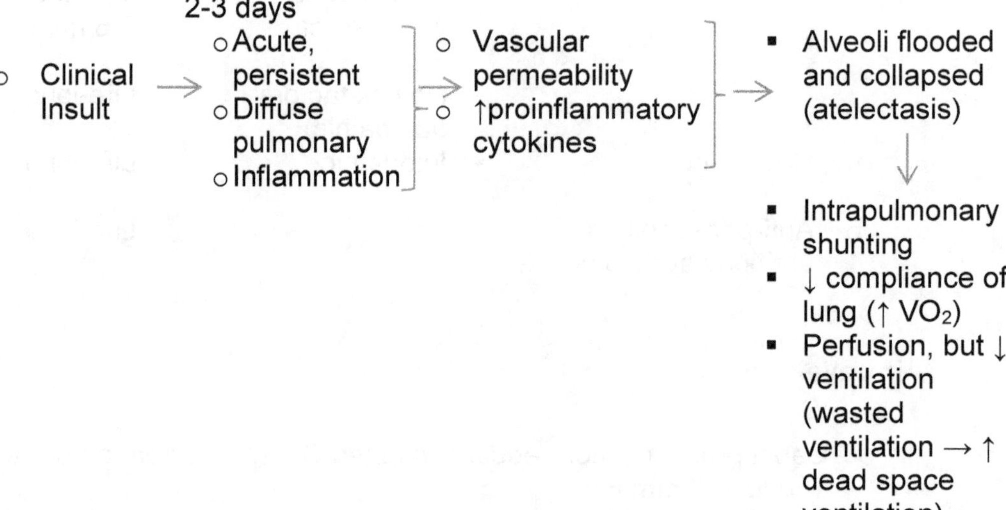

  - Severe in ARDS, hypoxemia may be associated with hypercapnia
    - ↑ VO_2 (↑ work of breathing)
    - ↑ dead-space ventilation
  - Respiratory failure explained by heart failure or volume overloads (these may co-exist with ARDS)

Range of severities

Severity	PO_2 / FI O_2 (PEEP of 5 cm H_2O) mm Hg	kPa
- Mild	201 to 300	26.7 to 39.9
- Moderate	101 to 200	13.4 to 26.6
- Severe	≤ 100	≤ 13.3

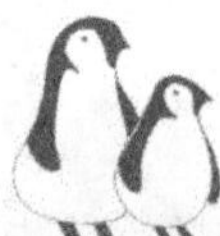

- Perform a focused physical examination for acute respiratory distress syndrome (ARDS).

Disorder	Cause
o Shock	- Any cause
o Sepsis	- Lung infections, other bacteremic or endotoxic states
o Trauma	- Hypotension, especially if prolonged, or with trauma - The systemic inflammatory response syndrome (SIRS) - Obstetric causes: amniotic fluid embolism, pre eclampsia - High altitude related lung injury - Head injury, lung contusion, fat embolism - Gastric, near-drowning, tube feeding, Inhaled- O2, smoke
o Aspiration	- Blood transfusions (especially if massive), leukoagglutinin,DIC (disseminated intravascular coagulation), thrombotic thrombocytopenic purpura - Pancreatitis, uremia - Narcotics, barbiturates, aspirin, “street drugs”
o Hematologic	- Chemicals-paraquat - Irritant gases- NO_2, CO_2, SO_2, NH_3 - Radiation, air embolism, altitude
o Metabolic	
o Drugs	
o Toxic	
o Miscellaneous	

- Appropriate setting
  - Pulmonary injury, shock, trauma
  - Acute event
  - Clinical respiratory distress, tachypnea

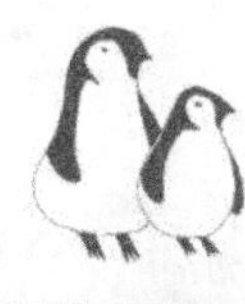

- o Diffuse pulmonary infiltrates on chest radiography
  - Interstitial or alveolar pattern (or both)
- o Hypoxemia
  - PaO_2/FiO_2 ratio <150
- o Exclude
  - Chronic pulmonary disease accounting for the clinical features
  - Left ventricular failure (most series require pulmonary artery wedge pressure <18 mm Hg)

Abbreviations: ARDS, Acute respiratory distress syndrome; BOOP, Bronchiolitis obliterans organizing pneumonia; COP, cryptogenic organizing pneumonia; FiO_2, fraction of inspired oxygen

Adapted from: Davey P. *Wiley-Blackwell* 2006, page 211; Ghosh AK. *Mayo Clinic Scientific Press* 2008, Table 4-14 and Table 4-15, page 159.

➢ Causes

- Give common causes of ARDS (acute respiratory distress syndrome).

o Lung	- Inhalation injury - Aspiration - Near drowning - Pneumonia - Lung trauma
o Systemic	- Sepsis - Trauma - Multiple blood transfusions - Pancreatitis

- Give the criteria to diagnose acute respiratory distress syndrome (ARDS), and to classify its degree of severity.

➢ Diagnostic criteria

- o Acute onset within 48 – 72 hr
- o Respiratory distress
  - $PO_2 / FI_{O2} \leq 300$ mm Hg
  - Bilateral alveolar infiltrates
- o PCW (pulmonary capillary wedge [pulmonary artery catheterization]) pressure < 18 mm Hg
- o No associated L-HF (left-sided heart failure; PCW pressure ≥ 18 mm Hg suggests cardiogenic pulmonary edema

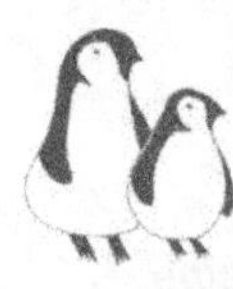

- Lung
- Shock
- Sepsis
- Pancreas
- Trauma
- Transfusion

- Infection
- Pancreatitis

➢ Grading

	Arterial PO_2 / FI_{O2} (mm Hg)
o Mild	200 - ≤ 300
o Moderate	100 - ≤ 200
o Severe	≤ 100

➢ Treatment

- Endotracheal tube, with delivery of ventilation by volume or pressure
  - Assist / control
    - Preset tidal volume or pressure
  - Pressure support for spontaneous breathing patients
  - Synchonized intermittent mandatory ventilation (SMV)
    - Preset rate and tidal volume
- In ARDs
  - Use O_2, mechanical ventilation plus PEEP
- Mechanical ventilation
- Possible mortality benefit with
  - Extracorporeal membrane oxygenation
  - Neuromuscular blockade
- No mortality benefit with inhaled vasodilators, corticosteroids, conservative volumes of fluids infused nursing in prone position
- Treat any associated cardiogenic edema from LV (left ventricle) systemic dysfunction
- Treat associated lung infection
- Note: mortality rate from all-cause ARDS is 40%, even higher with pneumonia and sepsis.

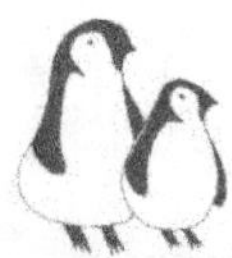

- Give the endpoints of PEEP (positive end-expiratory pressure) for the treatment of ARDS.

  - TV (tidal volume)
    - 6 mL/kg ideal body weight
  - End-inspiratory pressure
    - < 30 cm H_2O
  - Oxyhemoglobin saturation
    - 88% on an FI_{O2} of 60%
  - CVP < 4 mm Hg, or
  - PAO (pulmonary artery occlusion) pressure < 8 mm Hg

- Give the special considerations of mechanical ventilation and PEEP in ARDS.
  - Tidal volume
    - Calculate tidal volume from ileal (not actual) body weight
    - Use tidal volumes which are of modest value (6 mL/kg ideal body weight, not usual 12 mL/kg) to allow for hypoventilation of the alveoli with hypocapnia ("permissive hypercapnia") which may ↓ ventilator-induced lung injury

  - PEEP
    - Recruits collapsed alveoli
    - Benefit
      - ↑ compliance of lung
      - ↑ functional capacity
      - ↑ V /Q (ventilation/perfusion) matching
      - ↑ oxygenation
      - Avoid excessive PEEP (8 and not 15 cm H_2O), so as not to
      - ↓ venous return
      - ↑ pulmonary vascular resistance
      - ↓ CO (cardiac output)
      - ↓ BP (blood pressure)
      - ↓ barotrauma
      - ↓ pneumothorax

- Give the commonest chronic complication of recovery from an illness in the ICU, and its clinical Causes/associations.

  - ~75% of ICU survivors will have neurophychiatric impairment (acquired dementia), which correlates with mechanical ventilation and hypoxia, as well as glycemic control.

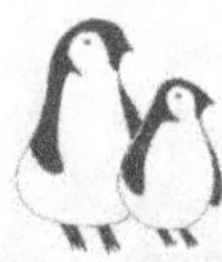

NON-INVASIVE POSITIVE-PRESSURE VENTILATION (NPPV)

- Definition
  - IPAP (Inspiratory positive airway pressure)
    - ↓ inspiratory effect
  - EPAP (end-expiratory positive airway pressure)
    - Recruits collapsed or flooded alveoli
    - ↓ work load from high airway resistance
  - Driving pressure of NPPV = IPAP – EPAP

- Major uses
  - COPD
  - Acute cardiogenic pulmonary edema (CPAP also useful)
  - Immunocompromised patient (to avoid intubation)
  - Following failed extubation in patients with chronic lung disease and hypercapnia
  - Possibly in selected patients with exacerbations of their asthma

- Uncooperative
- Unable to fit mask
- CNS
  - Sleepiness
  - Encephalopathy
  - Bulbar dysfunction
- ↑ secretions

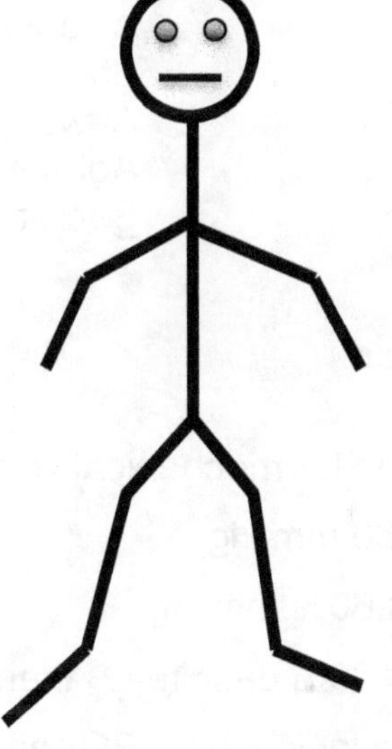

- Lung
  - Respiratory arrest
  - Upper airway obstruction
- Heart
  - Arrest
  - Shock
  - Hemodynamic instability
  - Arrhythmia

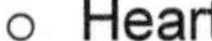

- Septic shock
- Severe acidosis
- GI
  - Upper GI bleeding
  - Nausea / vomiting

Clinical Caution

- If patient does not respond to 1-2 hr NPPV, consider intubation to prevent respiratory arrest.

- Give indications for considering the use of NPPV before mechanical ventilation, and the contraindications for NPPV.
  - Indications
    - Heart
      - Cardiogenic pulmonary edema
    - Lung
      - COPD exacerbation
      - In recently extubated patients (to present recurrence of need for mechanical intubation for respiratory failure)
      - Acute respiratory failure in immunosuppressed persons
  - Contraindications
    - AAS-AAS
      Arrest, respiratory
      Acidosis (pH < 7.10)
      Stability poor
      Airway protection not possible
      Agitated patient
      Secretions excessive

Mechanical Ventilation

- Give the indications for mechanical ventilation
  - Arterial PO_2 < 60 mm Hg
  - O_2 saturation < 60% mm Hg
  - O_2 saturation < 60% despite O_2 therapy
  - Note: use these indications (PO_2 and O_2% sat) regardless of arterial PCO_2

Setting the respiratory rate to high on a mechanical ventilator may cause air trapping (auto-PEEP) in the alveoli.

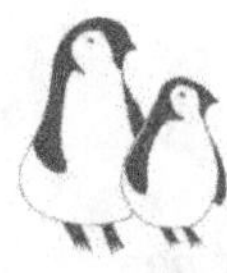

- Give the mechanisms for the development of auto-peep, and the findings on the ventilator flow tracing which will suggest this diagnosis.
    - Diagnosis
        - Continuous expiratory flow to point where inspiratory flow begins
        - Hypotension (↓ preload)
    - Mechanisms
        - ↑ resistance in airway
        - ↑ demand for ventilation
        - ↓ expiratory time

- Give the adjustments to the mechanical ventilator and the physiological endpoint for the following 3 clinical conditions.

Clinical condition	Adjustment to ventilator	Physiological endpoint
○ Respiratory acidosis	↑ RR (respiratory rate)	↓ $aPCO_2$
○ Respiratory alkalosis	↓ RR	↑$aPCO_2$
○ Tissue oxygenation	↑ FI_{O2} ↑ PEEP	↑aPO_2 ↑ O_2 saturation

Watch out for wrong answer temptation on MCQ

- When weaning a patient from mechanical ventilation, do not use synchronized intermittent mandatory ventilation.

"Success is not final, failure is not fatal:
It is the courage to continue that counts."
Winston Churchill

RESPIRATORY FAILURE

➢ Categorization of hypercapnia (↑PaO_2)

	Cause	EXAMPLE	VE	VD/VT	A-a gradient
o	Defective central control of breathing	- Drug overdose - Most causes of coma	↓	Normal	Normal
o	Neuro-muscular disease	- ALS - Spinal cord lesions - Myasthenia gravis - Guillian-Barre	↓	Normal or ↑	Normal or ↑
o	Chest wall disease	- Kyphoscoliosis - Large effusions	↓	Normal or ↑	Normal or ↑
o	Primary lung disease	- COPD	Normal or ↑	↑	↑

Abbreviations: ALS, amyotropic lateral sclerosis; COPD, chronic obstructive pulmonary disease; VE, minute ventilation; VD, dead space; VT, tidal volume

Permission granted: Davey P. *Wiley-Blackwell* 2006, page 198.

- Perform a focused physical examination for causes of disorder of ventilation.
  - o CNS lesions
    - Meningitis
    - Encephalitis
    - Stroke
    - Trauma
    - Anxiety, hysteria, pain
    - Raised intracranial pressure
  - o Brainstem
    - Amyotrophic lateral sclerosis
    - Post-paralytic condition
    - Overuse fatigue
    - CVA Respiratory centre depression
    - Hypercapnia
    - Brainstem injury
    - Spinal cord and PNS
    - Motor neuron disease (e.g., ALS, amyotrophic lateral sclerosis)
    - Atrophy
    - Gaillain-Barre syndrome
      - ▪ Acute inflammatory immune-mediated and often demyelating polyneuropathies, which may lead to respiratory failure and bulbar dysfunction (oropharyngeal weakness)
    - Myasthenic crisis triggered by
      - ▪ Infection
      - ▪ Drugs
      - ▪ Pregnancy
    - Lesion at C3 to C5
    - Neuropathy

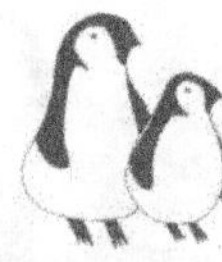

- Drugs
  - Rx causing ↓ cardiac output
  - Corticosteroids
  - Aminoglycosides
  - Salicylates, analeptics, adrenaline
  - Calcium channel blockers

- Lung
  - Kyphoscoliosis
  - Elevated diaphragm, emphysema
  - Pleural effusion
  - Pneumothorax
  - Obstruction in upper or lower respiratory tract
  - Atelectasis, pneumonia
  - Trauma
  - Pulmonary reflexes: irritant gases, atelectasis, pneumothorax
  - Ventilation
  - Duration of need for mechanical ventilation depends on function of diaphragm, intercostal and abdominal muscles

Hypercapnic Ventilatory Respiratory Failure

- Pathophysiology
  - Inadequate alveolar ventilation relative to CO_2 production
  - ↑ PCO_2 from
    - ↑ alveolar ventilation, +/-
      - ↓ respiratory drive
        - Drug
      - ↓ strength of respiratory muscles
      - Use mechanical ventilation, depending upon valves of VC [vital capacity]. MIP [maxima inspiratory pressure] and MEP [maximal expiratory pressure]
      - ↑ mechanical work of breathing (↑ VO_2)
      - ↓ gas exchange

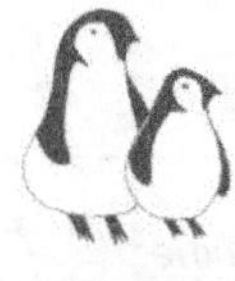

- Chest wall disorders (↓ chest movement)
  - Kyphoscoliosis
  - Rib fractures (pain)
  - Trauma
  - Flail chest
  - Respiratory muscle disease
  - Rupture, myopathy

- Muscular dysfunction
  - Muscular dystrophies
  - Guillain-Barre syndrome
  - Myasthenia gravis
  - Malnutrition
  - Acidosis
  - Hypoxemia
  - Anemia
  - Low cardiac output
  - Steroids
  - Post paralytic condition
  - Detraining, atrophy, overuse fatigue
  - Increased workload

- Metabolic
  - Hypo/hyperthyroidism
  - Increased metabolism
  - Metabolic alkalosis/acidosis
  - Hypotension
  - Malnutrition

Adapted from: Ghosh AK. *Mayo Clinic Scientific Press* 2008, Table 4-8, page 154 and Table 4.14 and 4.15, page 159; Burton JL. *Churchill Livingstone* 1971, page 24.

- Treatment

  - Where necessary, mechanical ventilation, plus

	Guillain-Barre syndrome	Myasthenic crisis
o Plasma pheresis, or	√	√
o IV immune globulin	√	√
o Corticosteroids	No	√

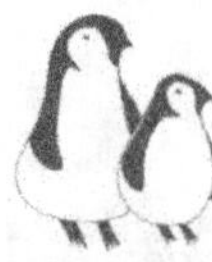

Hypoxemic Respiratory Failure

➢ Pathophysiology

- Give the pathophysiology of hypoxemic respiratory failure.

  - Alveolar dysfunction
    - Collapse
    - Fluid-filled (blood, edema, pus)

    } Perfusion, but ↓ ventilation (wasted ventilation → ↑ dead space)

    ↓

    ↓ arterial PO_2 (PCO_2 N / ↓)

  - Effective gas exchange requires adequate alveolar ventilation for the elimination of carbon dioxide, oxygen uptake across the alveolar-capillary membrane, and the delivery of oxygen to tissues.
  - *Hypoxemia* may result from the following:
    - Decrease in the inspired partial pressure of oxygen (e.g., at high altitude, including air travel or interruption of oxygen supply)
    - Hypoventilation
    - Ventilation-perfusion (V/Q) mismatch
    - Shunt
    - Diffusion barrier
  - Hypoxemia due to hypoventilation is characterized by an increased $PaCO_2$, decreased PaO_2, and a normal A-a gradient (estimation of the alveolar-arterial [A-a] gradient for oxygen is essential in analyzing the cause of hypoxemia).

Source: Ghosh AK. *Mayo Clinic Scientific Press* 2008, Table 4-7, page 153.

➢ Treatment
  - PEEP (positive end-expiration pressure; opens alveoli when are collapsed or flooded)
  - Note: hypoxemic respiratory is **not** treated with supplemental O_2 or mechanical ventilation, because the defect is intrapulmonary shunt physiology from collapsed or flooded alveoli.

- Give the diagnostic criteria for OHS (obesity hypoventilation syndrome).

  - Daytime arterial P co_2 > 45 mm Hg

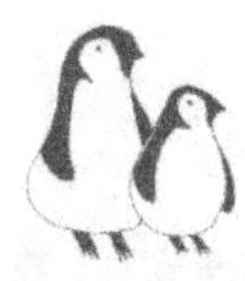

AMYOTROPHIC LATERAL SCLEROSIS (ALS)

- Types of motor neuron disease (degeneration of cortical motor neurons)
  - Frontal lobe of brain
    - Primary lateral sclerosis (PLS)
  - Anterior horn cells of spinal cord
    - Progressive muscular atrophy (PMA)
  - Combined cortical plus anterior horn cells
    - Amyotrophic lateral sclerosis

- Clinical features
  - Fasculations plus muscle weakness/atrophy
    - Spasticity
    - Clonus
    - N / ↑ reflexes
    - Bulbar symptoms
      - Respiratory insufficiency
      - Dysphagia
  - Onset
    - 80% cortical
      - Distal and asymmetrical
    - 20% bulbar

- Treatment
  - Supportive care
  - Riluzole
  - Assisted ventilation and feeding tube as needed

Pearls and Gems

- Motor neuron disease (MND) does **not**
  - Affect
    - Cognitive
    - Sensation
    - Eye muscle
  - Cause pain
- Fasciculations plus muscle weakness/atrophy suggests ALS
  - Fasciculations alone, or muscle weakness/atrophy alone do not suggest ALS

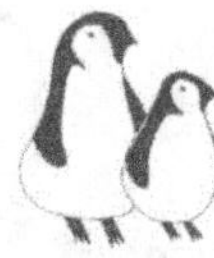

PNEUMOTHORAX

- Types
  - Primary
    - No associated lung disease (but subpleural blebs or bullae)
    - Tall male smokers
    - Cocaine use
    - Marfan syndrome
  - Secondary
    - COPD
    - CF
    - TB
    - Pneumocystis jirovecci

- What to think about on MCQs because of Pneumothorax.

Buzzwords	What "They" are Looking or
Young woman with lung disease and chylothorax or pneumothorax	Lymphangioleiomyomatosis
HIV infection	Pneumocystis jirovecci pneumonia
Interstitial lung disease	Langerhans cells histiocytosis

- Clinical

- Take a focused history for the causes of pneumothorax.
  - Traumatic
  - Iatrogenic
    - Thoracentesis
    - Thoracic surgery
    - Artificial pneumothorax
    - Cervical surgery, stellate block etc.
  - Spontaneous
    - Localized air space disorder
      - Congenital bullae
      - Localized emphysema
      - Acquired cysts
    - Generalized emphysema

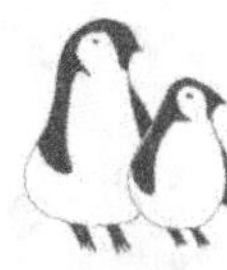

- Secondary to specific lung disease
  - Congenital
  - COPD (emphysematous bulla)
  - Diffuse cystic disease (CF)
  - Bronchiectasis; eosinophilic granuloma; tuberose sclerosis,
  - Silicosis

- Infection
  - TB
  - Lung abscess
  - Malignancy
  - Hydatid cysts

- Secondary to spontaneous mediastinal emphysema
  - Asthma
  - Labour
  - Straining at stool
  - Rapid decompression of divers

- Associated with menstruation
  - **Endometriosis**

Adapted from: Burton JL. *Churchill Livingstone* 1971, page 32; Baliga RR. *Saunders/Elsevier* 2007, page 287.

- Treatment
  - Iatrogenic
  - Primary
    - > 2 cm plus symptoms hospitalization O_2 needle thoracostomy chest tube
  - Secondary hospitalization, regardless of size, because of underlying lung disease
  - Prevention of recurrence
    - Thoracostomy
      - Repair plus pleurodesis (life-time recurrence, 5%)
      - Plus chemical pleurodesis (life-time recurrence, 25%)

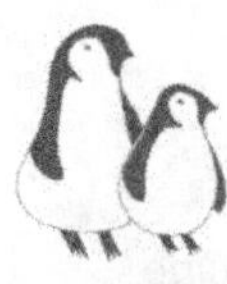

SLEEP APNEA SYNDROMES

- Sleep apnea syndromes may be either
  - Obstructive, associated with a "crowded pharynx" (large long soft palate) leading to upper airway obstruction during sleep
  - Central (associated with CNS disease or HF heart failure], or
  - Sleep-related hypoventilation syndrome

Obstructive Sleep Apnea (OSA)

- Definition
  - No airflow for ≥ 10 sec despite respiratory effect during sleep

- Terms

	↓ airflow
o Apnea	– Complete stopped
o Hypoapnea (aka disordered breathing event)	– Decreased

- Disordered breathing events = complete plus partial ↓ airflow
- Severity of OSA depends upon AHI:
  - AHI (apnea-hypoapnea; disordered breathing events per hour of sleep)

AHI	OSA
5 to 15	Mild
> 30	Severe

- Give a classification of OSA based on AHI (apnea-hypopnea index).

  - AHI (apnea-hypopnea index)
    - Number of apneas plus hypopneas per hour of sleep

Classification	AHI
– Mild	5-15
– Moderate	16-30
– Severe	> 30

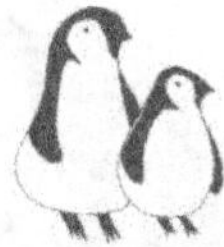

- Pathogenesis: Upper airways narrowing causing brief, repetitive cycles of repeated deoxygenation-reoxygenation
  - Primary
  - Secondary
    - ↑ BMI ("obesity)
    - Alcohol
    - Sedatives
    - Abnormal anatomy

▪ Jaw	– Micrognathia
▪ Tongue	– Macroglossia
▪ Tonsils	– Hypertrophy
▪ Mass	– Upper airway

- Clinical
  - Nocturnal hypoventilation
  - Nocturnal awakenings
  - Morning headaches
  - Daytime sleeping
- Complications

- Give complications of OSA which may be commonly underrecognized.

o CNS	– CVA – Mood disorders
o Heart	– CAD (coronary artery disease) – HF (heart failure) – MI (myocardial infarction) – AF (atrial fibrillation)
o Lung	– PAH (pulmonary artery hypertension) – Hypercapnic respiratory failure
o Endocrine	– Insulin resistance

- Diagnosis
  - Polynography

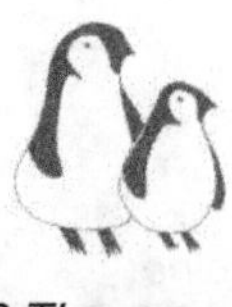

- Treatment
  - Associated/causative factors
    - Obesity
    - Alcohol
    - Sleeping
    - Drugs supine
  - Positive airway pressure
    - CPAP (continuous positive airway pressure)
    - BPAP (bilevel positive airway pressure: separate PAPs for inspiration and for expiration → pressure support to keep airways open and to improve alveolar hypoventilation
    - Autotitrating PAP machine
    - Nasal end-expiratory PAP
  - Correct anatomical abnormalities
    - Soft palate
    - UPPP (uvulopalatopharyngoplasty)
    - Mandible
      - Oral appliances
      - MMA (maxillomandibular advancement)
    - Tonsils
      - Tonsillectomy for hypertrophy of tonsils

- In the patient with insomnia and daytime sleepiness, give 2 conditions which can be diagnosed on polysomnography.
  - OSA (obstructive sleep apnea)
    - May be associated with obesity-hypoventilation syndrome (OHS)
  - Periodic leg movement disorder
    - May be associated with restless leg syndrome

- In the obese patient, who may also have COPD, and without a polysomnogram, give the laboratory test which helps to distinguish OSA from OHS (obesity-hypoventilation syndrome).
  - OHS is associated with
    - An awake ↑ PCO_2
    - Hypoventilate during REM (rapid eye movement) sleep

- Give 2 conditions which benefit from CPAP (continuous positive airway pressure).
  - OSA (obstructive sleep apnea)
  - OHS (obesity-hypoventilation syndrome)

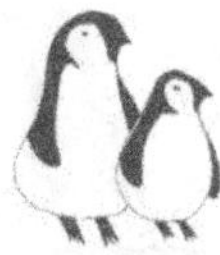

Central Sleep Apnea (CSA) **Syndrome**

- Pathogenesis
  - ↓ brainstem ventilation drive during non-REM sleep → no breathing for > 10 sec → ↑ arterial Pco_2 → ↑ ventilation → ↓ arterial Pco_2 to near the apneic threshold (no hypercapnia, as occurs with hypoventilation syndromes)
  - Brief, repetitive deoxygeneration
    - Reoxygenation cycles

- Causes

- Give causes of central sleep apnea (CSA) syndrome.

CNS	– CVA (cerebrovascular accidents) – Brainstem lesions
Heart	– HF (heart failure) – AF (atrial fibrillation)
Kidney	– Kidney failure
Drugs	– Opiates
CPAP	– CPAP-emerged CSA (aka complex apnea)

  - High altitude-related illness
  - Idiopathic

- Take a focused history and perform a focused physical examination for obstructive sleep apnea (aka Pickwickian Syndrome).

  - General
    - Daytime fatigue
    - Headache, particularly in the morning
    - Poor quality of life
  - Sleep
    - Daytime somnolence
    - Unrefreshing sleep
    - Snoring

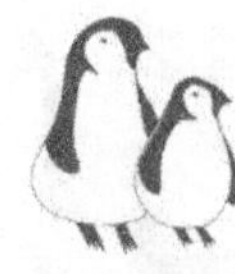

- CNS
  - Poor concentration
- Lung
  - Shortness of breath
- GI
  - Gastroesophageal reflux disease (GERD)
- Feet
  - Swelling of feet
- Family history
  - Obesity
- Physical examination
  - Habitus
  - Head and neck
  - Lung
  - CVS
    - R-HF
    - Pulmonary hypertension
    - Systemic hypertension

Adapted from: Baliga RR. *Saunders/Elsevier* 2007, pages 290 and 291.

- Treatment
  - Correct underlying/associated conditions
  - CPAP; if CPAP-emergent CSA develops, then use
  - ASV (adaptive seroventilation)
  - Supplemental
    - O_2
    - Low concentration CO_2
  - Acetazolamine
  - Theophylline
    - Monitor for dysarrhythmias

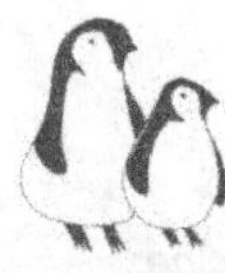

Sleep-Related Hypoventilation Syndrome (SRHS)

➢ Pathophysiology

- Give the changes in pulmonary physiology which distinguish OSA and CSA from SRHS.

Findings	OSA	CSA	SRHS
o Repetitive cycles of deoxygeneration (↓ oxyhemoglobin saturation) – reoxygenation	Brief	Brief	Sustained
o ↓ oxyhemoglobin saturation $< 90\%$ for ≥ 5 min $> 30\%$ of total sleep time	No	No	Yes
o Hypercapnia	No	No	Yes
o Mixed condition	N	No	Yes – may be associated with OSA or CSA

➢ Causes/associations

- o Obesity-associated hypoventilation syndrome (OHS)
  - Hypercapnia arterial $Pco_2 > 45$ mm Hg during daytime OHS may co-exist with OSA
    - → CPAP, or
    - → BPAP plus supplemental O_2
- o COPD
  - Muscle atonia during REM sleep → ↓↓ oxyhemoglobin saturation
  - Overlap of SRHA and OSA
- o Restrictive lung disease
- o Kyphoscoliosis, myxedema and many neuromuscular diseases (e.g., muscular dystrophy, cervical spine injury, myasthenia gravis and polio), by impairing the respiratory pump.

➢ Treatment

- o Underlying disease (e.g., COPD)
- o BPAP ± supplemental O_2

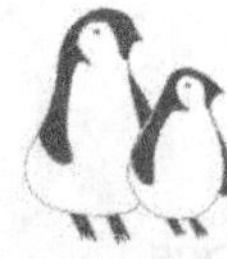

- Give the reason why and situations when BPAP +/- supplemental O_2 may be preferable to CPAP in SRHS (sleep-related hypoventilation syndromes) related to neuromuscular disease

  - CPAP may be sufficient for OSA when there is no impairment of the respiratory pump
  - When neuromuscular disease-associated SRHS (sleep-related hypoventilation syndrome) is associated with hypercapnia-associated reduction in respiratory drive, the treatment options include
    - BPAP +/- supplemental O_2
    - Tracheostomy plus home ventilation

- Give risk factors for the development of hypercapnic respiratory failure in the setting of hypoventilation syndromes.

  - Right-side heart failure (R-HF)
  - Pulmonary hypertension (PHT)
  - Polycythemia

Continuous Positive Airway Pressure (CPAP)

Nasal congestion from rhinitis is common with the use of CPAP (continuous positive airway pressure).

- Give the treatment for CPAP-associated nasal congestion.

  - In-line heated humidity with distilled water helps to prevent CPAP-associated rhinitis and nasal congestion

> "Always do your best. What you plant now, you will harvest later."
>
> Og Mandino

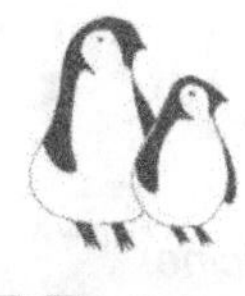

PULMONARY FIBROSIS

- Definition
  - Ideopathic fibrosing interstitial pneumonia

- Give a systematic approach to the causes of pulmonary fibrosis.

- Idiopathic
  - Acute respiratory distress syndrome/acute lung injury
  - Alveolar microlithiasis
  - Bronchiolitis obliterans with organizing pneumonia/cryptogenic organizing pneumonia (BOOP/COP)
  - Eosinophilic lung disease
  - Idiopathic pulmonary fibrosis- usual interstitial pneumonia (IPF-UIP)
  - Langerhans cell histiocytosis/eosinophilic granulomatosis
  - Lymphangioleiomyomatosis (LAM)
  - Lymphocytic interstitial pneumonia (LIP)
  - Non-specific interstitial pneumonia (NSIP)
  - Pulmonary alveolar proteinosis

- Idiopathic
  - Acute interstitial pneumonia
  - ARDS, acute respiratory distress syndrome
  - Pulmonary alveolar proteinosis
  - Respiratory bronchiolitis interstitial lung disease
- Congestion
- Infection
  - Bronchiectasis
  - Cystic fibrosis
  - Granulomatous diseases
    - Sarcoidosis
    - Wegener granuloma
  - Mycosis
  - Psittacosis
  - Tuberculosis
  - Varicella
- Infiltration
  - Alveolar cell carcinoma
  - Leukemia
  - Lymphangitis carcinomatosis

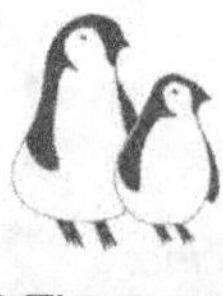

- Immune (collagen-vascular)
  - GS (Goodpasture syndrome)
  - PAN (polyarteritis nodosum)
  - Rheumatoid arthritis
  - Scleroderma
  - SLE (systemic lupus erythematosis)
  - WG, Wegener granulomatosis (granulomatosis with polyangiitis)
- Irradiation
- Toxins/drugs
  - Aluminium
  - Asbestos
  - Bagassosis
  - Benylum
  - Berglliosis
  - Busulphan
  - Byssinosis
  - Cadmium
  - China-clay
  - Chromium
  - Coal dust
  - Fumes
  - Iron
  - Irradiation
  - Kaolin
  - Nickel
  - Nitrofurantoin
  - Paraquat poisoning
  - Phenytoin
  - Silicon
  - Sulfonamides
  - Talc
  - Vomitus
- Hypersensitivity
  - "Hot tub" lung non-TB mycobacteria
  - Bird fancier lung
  - Chronic eosinophilic pneumonia (Farmers lung)
  - Farmer's lung reaction to Thermophilic actinomycetes (hay, grain farmers)
  - Mushroom workers lung
  - Paprika splitters lung
  - Pituitary snuff-taker's lung
  - Silo fillers disease
  - Workers in gas works
- Fibrosing Alveolitis
  - Rheumatoid lung
  - Desquamative interstitial pneumonitis
- Aspiration
- Histocytosis
  - Letterer-Siwe disease
  - Hand Schuller Christian disease
- Cardiac
  - Pulmonary edema
  - Mitral stenosis ossification

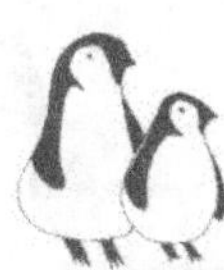

- Multiple pulmonary infarcts
- Uramic lung

- Neoplastic
  - Alveolar cell carcinoma
  - Lymphangitis carcinomatosa
- Lung
  - Pulmonary hemosiderosis
- Liver biliary cirrhosis
- Kidney
  - Goodpasture's syndrome
  - Alveolar proteinosis
  - Alveolar microlithiasis
- Drugs/toxins
  - Drugs e.g., amiodarone, bleomycin, methotrexate, phenytoin, sulfasalazine
  - Pneumoconiosis
    - Sand blasting
    - Asbestosis (↑ risk of mesothelioma)
- Tumour
  - Langerhans cell histiocytosis (eosinophilic granuloma, histiocytosis X)
- Miscellaneous
  - Wegner granulomatosis
  - Eosinophilic granuloma
  - LS disease
  - HSC disease
  - Good posture syndrome
  - Alveolar microlithiasis/ proteinosis
  - Pulmonary hemosiderosis

Abbreviation: HSC, Hand-Schuller-Christian disease; LS, Letterer-Siwe disease; PAN, polyarteritis nodosa; SLE, systemic lupus erythematosis

Adapted from: Davies IJT. *Lloyd-Luke* 1972, page 128; Burton JL. *Churchill Livingstone* 1971, page 29; Talley NJ, et al. *Maclennan & Petty Pty Limited* 2003, page 127; Ghosh AK. *Mayo Clinic Scientific Press* 2008, Table 23-11, page 917.

- Clinical
  - The physical signs of pulmonary fibrosis is the same as for collapse, but chest X-ray of collapse is usually homogenous, where as fibrosis is non-homogeneous.
  - Inspiratory basal crackles
  - Dullness of lung bases
  - Bronchial breathing

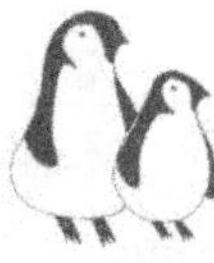

- Perform a focused physical examination to distinguish between the major causes of dullness at a lung base.
    - Pleural effusion: stony, dull note; trachea may be deviated to the opposite side in large effusions
    - Pleural thickening: trachea not deviated; breath sounds will be heard
    - Consolidation: vocal resonance increased; bronchial breath sounds and associated crackles
    - Collapse; trachea deviated to the affected side; absent breath sounds

Adapted from: Baliga RR. *Saunders/Elsevier* 2007, page 252.

- Give the characteristics and causes of bronchial breathing.
    - "blowing, gap, long expiration"
    - Associated with
        - Consolidation
        - Collapse
        - Cavity
        - Effusion
        - Pneumothorax

- Give 3 causes of dullness of the lung base not related to consolidation, cavitation or collapse.
    - Pleural effusion
    - Thickened pleura
    - Paralyzed hemidiaphragm

While IPF is characterized by a slow, progressive decline in pulmonary function, IPF may also be associated with acute exacerbations.

- Give the features which suggest an **acute exacerbation of IPF** (idiopathic pulmonary fibrosis).
    - Unexplained ↑, or new development of dyspnea in < 30 d
    - GGO (ground-glass opacity)
    - Consolidation

    on a background of usual CT demonstrated pneumonia, with no other diagnostic consolidation

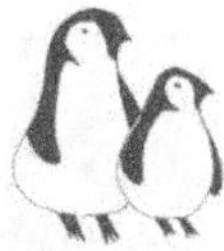

- Diagnostic imaging
    - Chest X-ray non-homogeneous collapse
    - The causes of lung collapse
        - Tumour
            - Bronchogenic carcinoma
            - Other intrabronchial tumours (e.g., bronchial adenoma)
    - Plugs
        - Asthma
        - Allergic bronchopulmonary aspergillosis
    - Infection
        - Extrinsic compression from hilar adenopathy (e.g., primary TB)
        - Tuberculosis

Adapted from: Baliga RR. *Saunders/Elsevier* 2007, page 292.

- High resolution CT (HRCT)

- Give the characteristic lung changes seen on diagnostic imaging in persons with idiopathic pulmonary fibrosis.

Pleura	- Subpleural cystic changes
Parenchyma	- Reticular opacitics - Traction bronchiectasis - Honeycomb appearance
Pattern	- Honeycomb - Reticular
Location	- Basal - Peripheral

- Preferential disinflation of lesions on chest X-ray
    - Upper lobe – TB, silicosis, pneumoconiosis
    - Lower lobe – bronchiectasis
    - Bilateral & symmetrical – pneumoconiosis

Clinical Gem

- Patient with IPF (idiopathic pulmonary fibrosis) do not benefit from intubation and mechanical ventilation (in-hospital mortality rate of ~ 90% with mechanical ventilation)

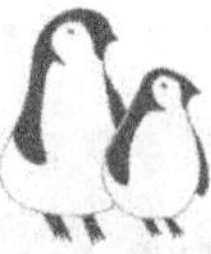

SO YOU WANT TO BE A PULMONARY PATHOLOGIST!

IPF (idiopathic pulmonary fibrosis) is partially a diagnosis of exclusion, but HRCT (high resolution CT) honeycomb or reticular pattern in the basal and peripheral portions of the lung are suggestive of this diagnosis (characteristic, but not specific). The same is the case for the pathology of IPF on lung biopsy.

- Give the features of IPF on lung biopsy.
  - Patchy and peripheral (subpleural) fibrosis → ↓ vascularity
  - Development of cysts → epithelial transformation → honeycomb/reticular appearance
  - Minimal
    - Inflammation
    - Ground-glass
- Ground-glass opacity is uncommon in IPF. Give the clinical significance of rapidly appearing ground-glass opacity.
  - Rapid appearance of ground-glass opacity in IPF suggests
    - Acute exacerbation
    - Infection
    - Pulmonary embolism

➢ Treatment
- Pulmonary rehabilitation
- O_2 therapy
- Management of complications/associations
  - PHT (pulmonary hypertension)
  - R-HF (right-sided heart failure, cor pulmonale)
  - OSA (obstructive sleep apnea)
  - Obesity
  - Emphysema
  - GERD (gastroesophageal reflux disease, with aspiration)
- Lung transplantation
- Note: no proven role for corticosteroids or immunosuppressants

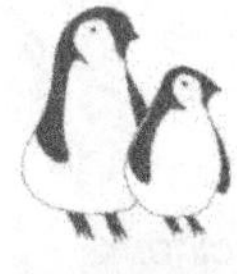

SARCOIDOSIS

- Definition
  - "...... a multisystem [non-caseating] granulomatous inflammatory disease of unknown cause.
  - An acute self-limited or a chronic multisystem disease of unknown cause resulting from noncaseating granulomas infiltrating organs.
  - Within the context of infiltration of tissues with noncaseating granulomas, give the characteristics of Lofgren syndrome
  - Lofgren syndrome is the acute, self-limited form of sarcoidosis
  - Lung involvement in 90%
  - Diagnosis of exclusion
  - May remit spontaneously
  - Low-dose corticosteroids may be useful

- Pathophysiology

- Give the current theory for the pathophysiology of sarcoidosis.
  - Sarcoidosis is "...... the end result of interactions among a persistent antigen, HLA class II molecules, and T-cell receptors" (Source: MKSAP 16 2013, Pulmonary, page 38).

- Give the sensitivity for the diagnosis of sarcoidosis with endobronchial ultrasound, with or without transbronchial biopsies.

Test	Sensitivity
Endobronchial ultrasound	85%
Endobronchial ultrasound plus transbronchial biopsies	95%

- Clinical

- Perform a focused physical examination for sarcoidosis.
  - General
    - Fever

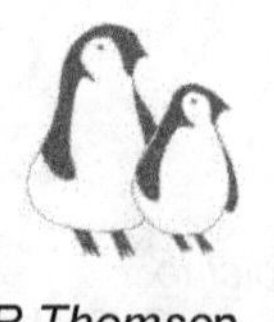

- CNS (may occur without signs elsewhere of sarcoidosis)
  - Neuropathy
    - Local deposit, or
    - Mononeuritis multiplex
  - Peripheral neuropathy
  - Lymphocytic meningitis (bilateral cranial nerve VII disease)
  - Diabetes insipidus
  - Mononeuritis multiplex
  - Cranial nerve palsies (meningeal infiltration)
- Eye
  - Uveitis
  - Ketatoconjunctivitis sicca
  - Sjogren syndrome
- Skin
  - Erythema nodosum
  - Non-specific infiltrates
  - Lupus pernio
- Lung
  - Bilateral hilar lymphadenopathy
  - Mottling of lung
  - Linear streaks
  - Pleural effusions do not occur
- Cardiac
  - Conduction defects
  - Valvular insufficiency
  - Cardiomyopathy
  - Cor pulmonale,
- Liver/spleen/nodes
  - Hepatosplenomegaly
  - Lymphadenopathy
  - Granuloma (in 86%)
  - Cholestasis
  - Post- necrotic cirrhosis
- Hematology
  - Spleen/nodes – granulomas
- Bone and joints
  - Cyst
  - Hypercalcemia
  - Terminal phalanges of hands
  - Arthralgia
  - Most common in ankles and knees. Axial skeleton spared.

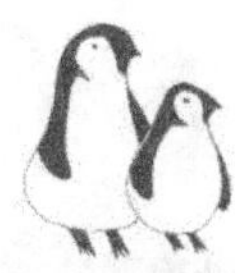

- Renal
  - Nephrolithiasis
  - Hypercalcemia
  - Nephrocalcinosis
  - Membrane nephropathy
- Endocrine
  - Thyroid nodules
  - Infertility
  - Hypogonadism

Adapted from: Talley N J, et al. *Maclennan & Petty Pty Limited* 2003, page 129-130; Davey P. *Wiley-Blackwell* 2006, pages 198 and 199.

- Give the skin manifestations of sarcoidosis.
  - Small, non-scaling, skin-coloured, dome-shaped papules, usually on face and neck
  - If lesions coalesce, nodules and plaque form on the trunk and extremities

Source: Baliga RR. *Saunders/Elsevier* 2007, page 437.

- In the context of sarcoidosis, give the meaning of the **Lofgren syndrome**, and the **Heerfordt syndrome**.
  - Lofgren
    - Fever
    - Arthralgia
    - Erythema nodosum
    - Hilar lymphadenopathy
  - Heerfordt
    - Fever
    - Uveitis
    - Parotid enlargement

➢ Diagnostic imaging

- Give the typical radiological features of silicosis.
  - Multiple nodules composed of concentric layers of fibrosis
  - Most prominent in upper lobes
  - Reticulation
  - Bullous emphysema
  - Pleural thickening

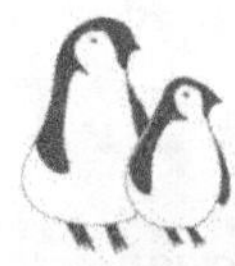

- Possible associated signs of
  - TB
  - Hilar adenopathy
- Complications of
  - Corpulmonale
  - Pneumothorax

- Pneumoconiosis
  - Fibrosis of lungs due to dust
  - Focal emphysema
  - Progressive massive fibrosis
    - Especially in upper lobes
    - Often cavitate and calcify
  - Often progresses to cor pulmonale

Useful background: Grading of sarcoidosis

Grade	Abnormality (% cases)	% Resolution
0	Normal	-
1	BHL (65%)	80%
2	BHL and pulmonary infiltrate (22%)	50%
3	Pulmonary infiltrate without BHL (13%)	25%

Abbreviations: BHL, Bilateral hilar lymphadenopathy

Source: Davey P. *Wiley-Blackwell* 2006, page 198.

Trick Question

You are given a patient with multisystem disease, with fever, erythema nodosum, uveitis, hypercalcemia, and bilateral hilar lymphadenopathy. You are told that the man worked making light bulbs and semiconductors. You are thinking that the diagnosis is sarcoidosis, and that the occupational history is simply a "red herring" meant to distract you from the correct diagnosis.

- Give the occupational toxicity which may mimic sarciodosis.
  - Beryllium exposure

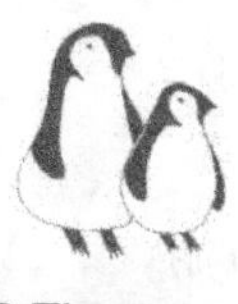

SO YOU WANT TO BE A RHEUMATOLOGIST!

The diagnosis of sarcoidosis may be suggested by ↑ serum angiotensin-converting enzyme levels, but this is not specific for the diagnosis. The diagnosis is made by biopsing any of the affected organs, except for the area of skin affected by erythema nodosum.

- Give the reason why skin biopsy from an area of erythema nodosum (EN) fails to help to secure the diagnosis in the patient with suspected sarcoidosis.
    - Tissue affected by sarcoidosis demonstrate noncaseating granulomas, suggestive of the diagnosis.
    - However, the biopsy of the skin from an area of EN will only demonstrates non-specific septal panniculitis.

- Treatment
    - Acute self-limited
        - NSAIDs
        - Corticosteroids
    - Joint pain, longer term
        - Hydroxylchlroquine
        - Colchicine
        - Methotrexate
    - If treatment with NSAIDs or corticosteroids fail
        - Sulfasalazine

- Give the findings on chest X-ray which suggest pleural thickening.
    - Hazy, homogeneous, poorly defined opacity
    - Opacity not confined to one lobe
    - On lateral view – looks smaller because of comparative decrease in thickness when seen in profile.
    - Screening – suggests pleural involvement
    - Associations – fibrosis, or collapse of underlying lung

Remember: The physical findings in pulmonary fibrosis are the same as in collapse.

Non-Specific Interstitial Pneumonia

- o One of the idiopathic diffuse parenchymal lung disease
- o Basal, ground glass on HRCT, with no honeycomb
- o Marked inflammatory infiltration
  - Lymphocytes
  - Plasma cells
- o Patchy deposit of collagen
- o R/o (rule out) associated connective tissue disease
- o Treat with tapering doses of corticosteroids +/- immunosuppression

BOOP and COP

- ➢ Terms
  - o BOOP
    - Bronchiolithis obliterans organizing pneumonia, caused by
      - ▪ Infection
      - ▪ Drugs
      - ▪ Collagen-vascular (connective tissue) disorders
  - o COP (cryptogenic organizing pneumonia) is the idiopathic form of BOOP

- ➢ Clinical
  - o Presents like a pneumoniawhich does not clear for 3-6 mon

- ➢ Chest X-ray
  - o Bilateral diffuse alveolar opacities
  - o Focal consolidation
  - o Multiple large nodules/masses, ½ found in periphery

- ➢ Treatment
  - o Tapering doses of corticosteroids for initial and for recurrent attacks

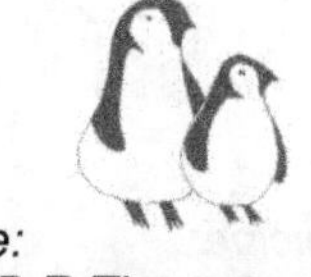

EXTRINSIC ALLERGIC ALVEOLITIS (Hypersensitivity Pneumonitis)

- Definition
  - Repeated exposure to antigens (e.g., moldy hay, thermophilic actinomycetes, bird feature) leads to acute, subacute or chronic lung disease localized mainly in upper- and middle-lung areas
  - Appears initially on HRCT as ground-glass centribular nodules, then progress to
    - Honeycomb appearance
    - Reticular lines
    - Traction bronchiectasis
  - Obstruction or restrictive defects seen on pulmonary function testing

- Causes/associations

- Give the causes of pulmonary eosinophilia and vasculitis

  - Lung
    - Asthma
    - ABPA
    - Chronic eosinophilic pneumonia
  - Drugs
  - Infection
    - Parasites
    - Loffler Syndrome (eosinophilia transient CXR infiltrate lasting 4-6 weeks, often related to bugs, parasites or worms)
  - Connective tissue disorders

Abbreviations: ABPA, Allergic bronchopulmonary aspergillosis; CXR, Chest x-ray

Adapted from: Davey P. *Wiley-Blackwell* 2006, page 204.

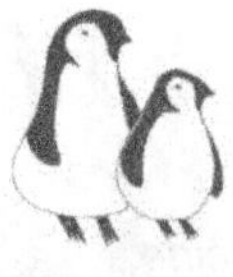

➢ Differential

- Give the distinction between acute and chronic extrinsic allergic alveolitis (EAA).

	Acute	Chronic
o WBC, ESR	– Ground glass	– May be normal
o Chest x ray	– Multiple nodules	– Fibrosis
o CT chest		– Fibrosis
o ABG	– Type 1 respiratory failure	
o Lung function tests	– Restrictive defect	– 50-60%
o Steroid response	– 80-90%	– Very poor
o Prognosis	– Very good	– Poor

Abbreviations: ABG, Arterial blood gases; EAA, Extrinsic allergic alveolitis

Source: Davey P. *Wiley-Blackwell*, 2006, page 200.

Pulmonary eosinophilic disorders

➢ Causes

- o Löffler syndromes
- o Transient pulmonary infiltrates
  - Peripheral eosinophilia
  - Associated with
    - ▪ Parasitic infections
    - ▪ Drug allergies
    - ▪ Exposure to inorganic chemicals (such as nickel carbonyl)
- o Eosinophilia in asthmatics
  - The most common cause is allergic bronchopulmoanry aspergillosis
- o Tropical eosinophilia which is secondary to filarial infection (*Wuchereria bancrofti* or *W. malayi Brug*)
- o Course is benign and respiratory failure almost unknown
- o Churg Strauss syndrome
  - Diagnosis requires four of the following features

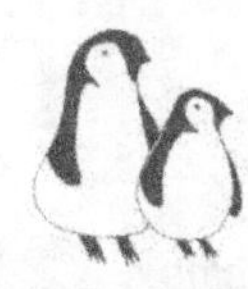

- Mononeuropathy or polyneuropathy
- Paranasal sinus abnormality
- Non-fixed pulmonary infiltrates visible on chest x-ray
- Blood vessels with extravascular eosinophils found on biopsy
- Asthma
- Eosinophilia greater than 10%
- ↑ IgE
- pANCA (positive in 50%)
- Pleural effusion
- Vasculitis on biopsy (multisystem disease)

- Eosinophilic pneumonia
  - Segmental bilateral peripheral ground glass infiltrates on CT
  - Restrictive lung function
- Hypereosinophilic syndrome
  - Eosinophilia <20 x 10^9/L
  - Pulmonary infiltrates and effusions
  - Myocardial infiltration and CHF

- Chronic eosinophilia pneumonia
  - Chronic debilitating illness characteristical malaise, fever, weight loss and dyspnea. The chest radiograph shows a peripheral alveolar filling infiltrate predominantly in the upper lobes (the graphic negative [opposite] of pulmonary edema)

Source: Baliga RR. *Saunders/Elsevier* 2007, page 273.

Fibrosing Alveolitis

- Causes
  - Primary
  - Secondary
    - Rheumatoid arthritis
    - Systemic lupus erythematosus
    - Scleroderma
    - Dermatomyositis
    - Chronic extrinsic allergic alveolitis

Source: Davey P. *Wiley-Blackwell* 2006, page 202.

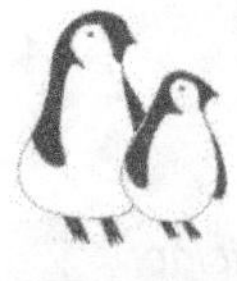

➢ Clinical

- Take a directed history and perform a focused physical examination for fibrosing alveolitis.

- History
    - Progressive exertional dyspnea (90%)
    - Chronic cough (74%)
    - Arthralgia/arthritis (19%)
    - Obtain a drug history (amiodarone, nitrofurantoin and busulfan)

- Physical examination
    - Chest
        - Bilateral, basal, fine, end-inspiratory crackles which disappear or become quieter on leaning forwards
        - The “velco-like” crackles do not disappear on coughing (unlike those of pulmonary edema)
        - Tachypnea (in advanced cases)
    - Hands (for rheumatoid arthritis, systemic sclerosis) - Clubbing
    - Face (for typical rash of SLE, heliotropic rash of dermatomyositis, typical facies of systemic sclerosis, lupus pernio of sarcoid)
        - Central cyanosis
    - Mouth (for aphthous ulcers of Crohn disease, dry mouth of Sjögren syndrome)
    - CVS
        - Signs of pulmonary hypertension: ‘a’ wave in the JVP, left parasternal heave and P_2
    - Examine patient for conditions which have similar pulmonary changes
        - Rheumatoid arthritis, SLE, dermatomyositis, chronic active hepatitis, ulcerative colitis, systemic sclerosis
        - Pneumoconiosis
        - Granulomatous disease; sarcoid, TB
        - Chronic pulmonary edema
        - Radiotherapy
        - Lymphangitis carcinomatosa
        - Extrinsic allergic alveolitis: farmer’s lung, bird fancier’s lung

Adapted from: Baliga RR. *Saunders/Elsevier* 2007, page 281; McGee SR. *Saunders/Elsevier* 2007, Box 27-2.

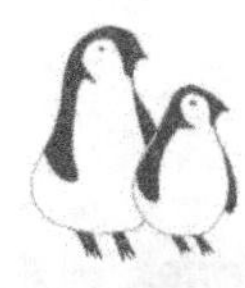

- Investigations

Useful background: Investigations to distinguish between acute and chronic Fibrosing Alveolitis

	Acute	Chronic
○ Lung function test defect	- Restrictive defect	▪ Restrictive defect
○ Chest x ray	- Ground glass	▪ Honeycomb
○ CT scan	- 'Alveolitis'	▪ 'Fibrosis'
○ ABG	- Type 1 failure	▪ Early: normal at rest, ↓ pO_2 on exercise ▪ Late: type I failure
○ RF/ANA		▪ 30-50%

Abbreviations: RF/ANA, Rheumatoid factor/antinuclear antibody; ABG, arterial blood gases

Source: Davey P. *Wiley-Blackwell* 2006, page 202.

"The price of greatness is responsibility."
Winston Churchill

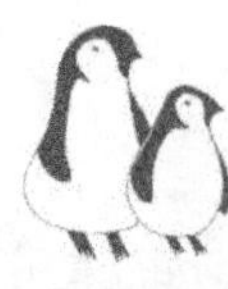

DIFFUSE PARENCHYMAL LUNG DISEASE (DPLD) **AND INTERSTITIAL LUNG DISEASE** (ILD)

- Terminology

	Portion of Lung Affected
o DPLD (diffuse parenchymal lung disease)	- Distal parenchyma
o ILD (interstitial lung disease)	- Distal parenchyma - Airways - Vessels - Pleura

- Demography
  - > 100 types of DPLD
  - Idiopathic in ~ 1/3
  - Prevalence $70/10^5$
  - Clinical progressive worsening of cough and dyspnea for > 3 mon, with diffuse changes on HRCT (high resolution CT)

- Causes

- Give causes of acute onset (A3, B, D2V) → and 20 causes of gradual onset DPLD.

  - Acute
    - A3 acute pneumonia / pneumonitis
      - Eosinophilic
      - Hypersensitivity
      - Interstitial (AIP)
    - B
      - Bronchiotitis obliterans organizing pneumonia (BOOP)
    - D2
      - Drug-induced pneumonitis
      - Diffuse alveolar hemorrhage syndrome
    - V
      - Vasculitis

-

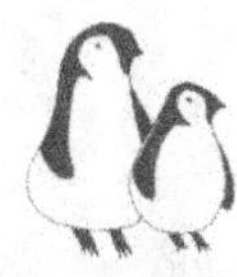

- o Gradual onset (much more common)

  - Idiopathic
    - ▪ Idiopathic pulmonary fibrosis (IPF)
    - ▪ Idiopathic DPLD
      - Cryptogenic organizing pneumonia (COP), the idiopathic form of BOOP [bronchiolitis obliterans organizing])
      - Interstitial pneumonia
      - Non-specific Lymphocyte
      - Acute (aka as idiopathic diffuse alveolar damage, or Hamman-Rich syndrome)

  - Inflammation / immune
    - ▪ RA (rheumatoid arthritis)
    - ▪ SSc (systemic sclerosis)
    - ▪ Polymyositis
    - ▪ Sarcoidosis
    - ▪ Acute/chronic eosinophilic
    - ▪ Pulmonary alveolar proteinosis

ACUTE INTERSTITIAL PNEUMONIA (aka IDAD [idiopathic diffuse alveolar damage], or Hamman-Rich syndrome)

➢ Causes/associations

- Give the causes of ARDS (acute respiratory distress syndrome).
  - Pneumonia
  - Sepsis
  - Inhalation damage
  - Drug/toxins
  - o Pneumoconiosis
    - Asbestosis
    - Coal
    - Silicosis
  - o Smoke
    - Histiocytosis (Langerhans cell histiocytosis)
    - Respiratory bronchiolitis interstitial lung disease
    - Desquamative interstitial pneumonia

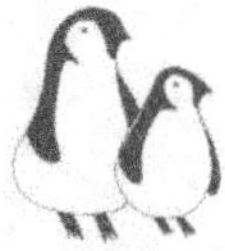

- Drugs
  - Chemotherapy
  - Amiodarone
  - Nitrofurantoin
- Toxins
  - Cocaine
  - Ammonia
  - Zinc chloride

SO YOU (REALLY REALLY) WANT TO BE A PULMONOLOGIST!

- Give the name of the inherited condition with involvement of the CNS and skin which has lung findings similar to a rare cause of DPLD (diffuse parenchymal lung disease). Oh my gosh – what trivia !!
  - Tuberous sclerosis has CNS and skin changes, plus pulmonary features similar to pulmonary lymphangioleiomyomatosis.

- Clinical
  - Rapid onset of symptoms, progressing to hypoxemic respiratory failure
  - Exclude other causes rapid onset DPLD A3, B, D2, V
    - Acute pneumonia/pneumonitis
      - Eosinophilic
      - Hypersensitive
      - Interstitial (AIP, acute interstitial pneumonia)
    - B
      - Bronchiolitis obliterans organizing pneumonia (BOOP)
    - D2
      - Drug-induced pneumonitis
      - Diffuse alveolar hemorrhagic syndromes
    - V1
      - Vasculitis
- Diagnosis
  - HRCT (high-resolution CT)
    - Pattern
    - Distribution
  - From the pattern and distribution of pulmonary changes on HRCT (not standard chest X-ray), the cause of the diffuse parenchymal lung disease (DPLD) may be suspected.

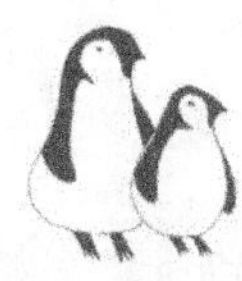

- Pattern
  - Septal – ↑ lymphatics e.g., Pulmonary edema, Lymphangitic cancer
  - Nodular – Sarcoidosis (small [< 1 cm] round lesion in the interstitium)
  - Reticulonodular
    - Sarcoidosis
    - Histiocytosis (pulmonary Langerhans cell histiocytosis)
    - Lymphangitic carcinomatosis
  - Ground-glass – Desquamative interstitial pneumonia
  - Honeycomb – Thick septal lines near cystic area (cystic area with epithelial transformation) at periphery of lung, suggestive of IPF (idiopathic pulmonary fibrosis)
  - Reticular – Suggestive of IPF
  - Consolidation – No specific cause of DPLD is suggested

– Note: About 20% of persons with chronic cough and dyspnea, plus a normal chest X-ray, will have DPLD seen on HRCT.

"With the new day comes new strength and new thoughts."

Eleanor Roosevelt

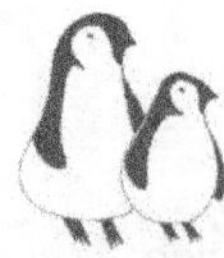

- Distribution (predominant area)

Suggestive diagnosis	Pattern	Distribution
o IPF	– Honeycomb – Reticular	▪ Basal ▪ Peripheral
o Sarcoidosis	– Nodular – Reticulonudular	▪ Upper lobe ▪ Central
o Hypersensitivity pneumonitis		▪ Mosaic ▪ Upper lobe

o Upper lobe
- Sarcoidosis
- Hypersensitivity pneumonitis

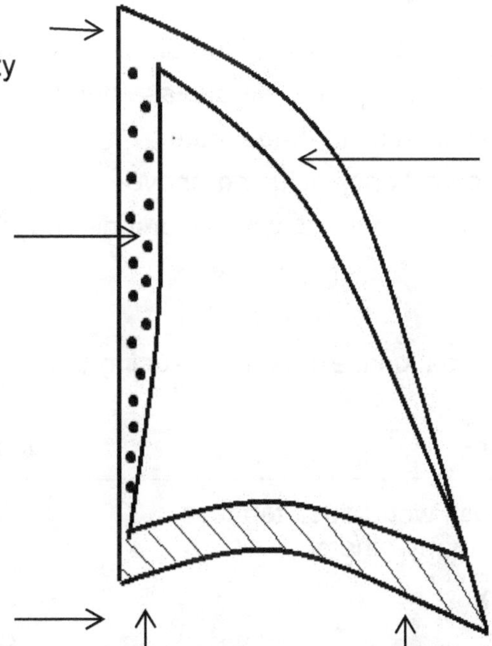

Sarcoidosis

➢ Hypersensitivity pneumonitis

➢ Mosaic pattern
  - o Pulmonary vasculitides
  - o Hypersensitivity pneumonitis
  - o RBAILD

o Basal
- IPF
- NSIP
- Asbestos

Central
- Sarcoidosis
- PAP

Peripheral
- IPF
- CEF
- COP

Abbreviations: CEP, chronic eosinophilic pneumonia; COP, cryptogenic organizing pneumonia; IPF, idiopathic pulmonary fibrosis; NSIP, non-specific interstitial pneumonia; PAP, pulmonary alveolar proteinosis; RBAILD, respiratory bronchiolitis-associated lung disease

- Treatment
  - ICU, mechanical ventilation, on TV (tidal volume)
  - Unproven benefit of corticosteroids
  - 50% mortality
  - May relapse or progress to chronic interstitial lung disease

OCCUPATIONAL LUNG DISEASE

- Types
  - Asthma, occupational
  - DPD (diffuse parenchymal lung disease), hypersensitivity pneumonitis
  - Pneumoconiosis (restrictive disease due to inhalation of mineral dust)
  - Toxic inhalation syndrome, acute
  - De novo conditions, including above
  - Occupational exposure, which worsens underlying lung disease
- Causes

- Give the occupational exposures causing 5 different types of lung disease.

Exposure	Lung disease
Grain dust, wood dust, tobacco, pollens, many others	Asthma
Asbestos	Pleural mesothelioma
Coal	Pneumoconiosis
Sandblasting and quarries	Silicosis
Industrial dusts	Chronic bronchitis
Birds	Psittacosis
Cotton	Byssinosis

Source: Filate W, et al. *The Medical Society, Faculty of Medicine, University of Toronto* 2005, Table 3, page 283.

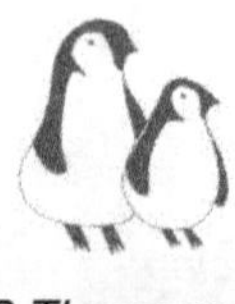

- Treatment
  - Identifying irritant
  - Remove person from exposure
  - Consider referral to specialist to optimize possible compensation lung disease

Asbestosis-Associated Lung Disease

- Pathophysiology
  - Inhalation of hydrated silicate fiber
  - Fiber deposited at bifurcations of airways taken up into interstitium of alveolar cells
  - Mechanism of pleural plaques, thickening etc. is unknown
- Pathology

- Give the pathology of the lung which suggests asbestosis.
  - Mesenchymal cells
    - Chronic inflammation
    - Proliferation
  - Fibrosis
  - ↓ alveolar-capillary units
  - Atelectasis
  - Formation of mass-like lesion

- Diagnostic imaging

- Give the characteristic lung changes seen on diagnostic in persons with asbestosis-associated lung disease.
  - Pleura
    - Plagues
      - Localized
      - Partially calcified
    - Thickening
    - Effusion
  - Parenchyma
    - Bilateral interstitial fibrosis

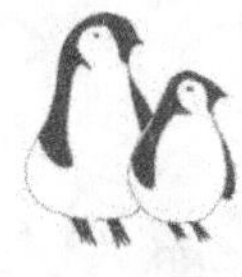

- Atelectasis
  - Single or multiple masses
  - Chest CT shows comet-tail appearance from hilum to base of lung
- Tumour
  - Mesothelioma
    - Pleural-based
      - Thickening
      - Nodular infiltrates
  - Cancer (especially smoking and asbestos exposure)

- Affects pleura and parenchyma of lung
  - Pleura
    - Localized, partially calcified plaque
    - Thickening
    - effusion
    - Cancer, mesothelioma
  - Parenchyma
    - Asbestos
    - Cancer
      - Small cell
      - Non-small cell
      - Mesothelioma

      } ↑ risk in smokers plus asbestosis exposure
- Asbestosis
  - One of the asbestos-associated lung disease

Silicosis

- Definition
  - A spectrum of diseases caused by inhalation of quartz (silica, crystalline silicon dioxide)
- Clinical
  - Lung disease
    - Acute
    - Chronic
    - Accelerated
    - ↑ risk
      - TB
      - Cancer
  - ↑ risk of autoimmune disease

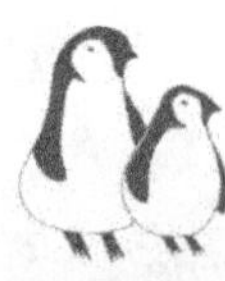

ANGIODEMA

- Pathophysiology
  - Angioedema may be mediated by mast cells or by the release of bradykinin.
  - **Mast-cell mediated** angioedema is triggered by
    - Allergies to food (e.g., peanuts, shrimp)
    - Drugs (NSAIDs, opiates)
    - Sensitivity to food additives
    - Articarial vaculitis
  - **Bradykinin-mediated** angioedema may be
    - Hereditary
    - Associated with
      - lupus
      - lymphoma
      - monoclonal gammopathy of underdetermined significance
      - use of ACE inhibitors
  - Mast-cell mediated ("allergic") angioedema may require urgent treatment.
    - Urgent
      - Epinephrine
      - IM; IV nebulized for nasal intake
    - Routine
      - Antihistamine
      - Corticosteroids

- Differential

- Give a simple clinical and laboratory way to differentiate between mast-cell mediated ("allergic") and bradykinin-mediated angioedema.

Finding	Mast Cell	Bradykinin-Mediated
o Angioedema	+	+
o Urticaria	+	-
o Bronchospasm	+	-
o Hypotension	+	-
↓ serum CI inhibitor, and ↓ serum C4 concentrations	-	+

- Treatment
  - Urgent
    - FFP (fresh fresh frozen plasma)
  - Routine
    - Short-term
      - IV C1 inhibitor (esterase) concentrate
    - Long-term: Danzole

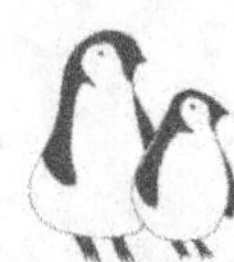

LYMPHAGIOLEIOLEIOMYOMATOIS (LAM)

- Clinical

- Give the typical clinical profile of the person who should be suspected as having LAM (leiomyomatosis).
    - Diagnosis of tuberous sclerosis, or
    - Young woman who develops pneumothorax or chylothorax, with chest x-ray also demonstrating hyperinflation.

- Causes
    - Molecular biology
        - Inactivating mutations of the TSC (tuberous sclerosis complex) gene activate the mTOR (mammalian target cells the parenchyma of the lung)
    - Evidence that LAM is a low-grade metaplastic neoplasm
        - LAM is a progressive pulmonary disease for which lung transplantation may be necessary
        - LAM may recur in the transplanted lung, suggesting that it may be a low-grade neoplastic condition which selectively targets the lung

- Diagnosis
    - VEGF-D (vascular endothelin growth factor – D) is increased in LAM, helping to distinguish LAM from other cystic lung conditions

"People must be retire at age 65, to have enough time to wait for their public Health Care!"

Grandad

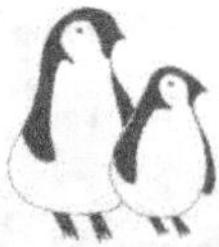

PARENCHYMAL LUNG DISEASE

- **Radiation-induced**

➢ Radiation pneumonitis
  - Occurs ~ 6 wk after exposure
  - Usually resolves ~ 6 mon after exposure
  - Affected area
    - Radiated area
    - Curiously, sometimes outside the radiation area
  - May improve with corticosteroids

- **Drug-induced**

  ➢ Methotrexate-associated Lung Disease

The immunosuppressant methotrexate is commonly used in gastrointestinal and rheumatology condition.

- Give the changes in the peripheral blood,high resolution CT (HRCT) and biopsy in persons with methotrexate-associated lung disease.

  - Peripheral blood eosinophilia in ~ 2/3
  - Diagnostic patterns
    - Diffuse reticular
    - Grand-glass
    - Consolidation
  - Pathology
    - Interstitial pneumonitis
    - Bronchiolitis obliterans organizing pneumonia
    - Diffuse alveolar damage
    - Fibrosis

SO YOU WANT TO BE A PULMONOLOGIST!

- Give types of lung damage associated with the use of amiodarone.
  - Parenchyma
    - Pneumonia
    - Pneumonitis
    - Fibrosis
  - Alveoli-diffuse damage
    - Hemorrhage
  - Pleura
    - Subpleural masses

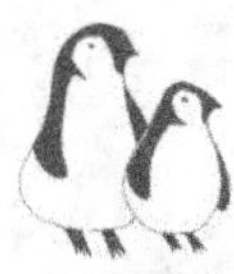

Smoking-Associated Parenchymal Lung Disease

- Pulmonary function testing

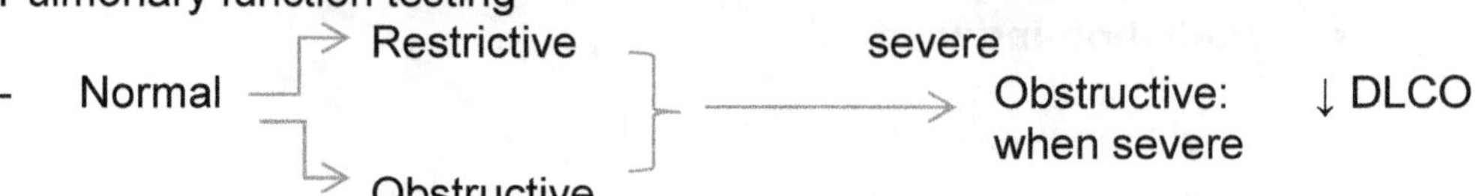

- HRCT
  - Range of changes, even when early, of
    - Bronchiolitis-associated lung disease (centrilobular micronodular disease)
    - Desquamative interstitial pneumonia (ground gall opacities)
    - Langerhans cell histiocytosis (upper lung cysts with nodules)

Organophosphate Poisoning

- Poisoning may be intentional or unintentional, and occur with drugs or chemicals

➢ Clinical

Excessive exposure to fertilizers containing organophosphates will increase activity of acetylcholinesterase, increase acetylcholine effects and cause a clinical syndrome.

Eyes	– Lacrimation – Miosis
Mouth	– Salivation
GI	– Vomiting – Diarrhea
GU	– Urination
Lung	– Bronchospasm

SLUDGE	or	DUMBELS
Salivation		Diarrhea
Lacrimation		Urinary
Urination		Miosis
Diarrhea		Bronchospasm
GI upset		Emesis
Emesis		Lacrimation
		Salvation

Aide de memoire have been offered in Board Basics page 299

- Treatment
  - Thankfully, organophosphate poisoning is not common, but it is important to recognize because there are specific antidotes. Treatment includes:
  - General measures ventilation, as needed removal of toxin from skin ("external decontamination")
  - Antidotes
    - Atropine
    - Pralidoxime
      - if CNS toxicity develops from atropine
    - Benzodiazepines
      - if convulsions develop

- In the context of organophosphate poisoning, give the features of atropine toxicity.
  - Fever
  - CNS toxicity
    - Delirium
    - Convulsions

Carbon Monoxide Poisoning

- Following a fun BBQ in the backyard, the host develops headache, light headedness, confusion and chest pain. Because of the exposure to smoke from BBQ, carbon monoxide (CO) poisoning is suspected, and the blood carboxyhemoglobin level is increased to 30%. However, the pulse oximetry reading was normal. Does the person have CO poisoning?
  - Yes, the carboxyhemoglobin concentration > 25% indicates severe CO poisoning.
  - Pulse oximetry measures both oxyhemoglobin and carboxyhemoglobin, and does not differentiate an elevated carboxyhemoglobin, and so is not useful to make the diagnosis of CO poisoning.

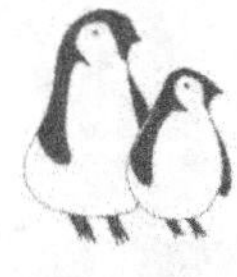

The care of the patient with poisoning is supportive, but **antidotes** are available for some drugs and chemicals.

- Give the antidote for the following.
    - Acetaminophen
    - Amphetamines
    - Amanitaphaloid mushrooms
    - Benzodiazepines
    - β-adrenergic blockers (BBs)
    - Calcium channel blockers (CCBs)
    - Digoxin
    - Heparin
    - Narcotics
    - Organophosphates
    - Tricyclic anti-depressants

If you have any difficulty finding all the antidotes, refer to a general textbook of Internal Medicine, or a review source such as Board Basics 2013, page 300-301.

"Optimism is the faith that leads to achievement.
Nothing can be done without hope and confidence."

Helen Keller

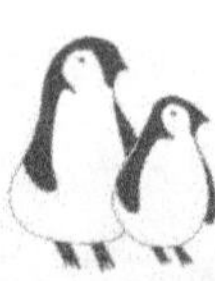

CLINICAL ANATOMY

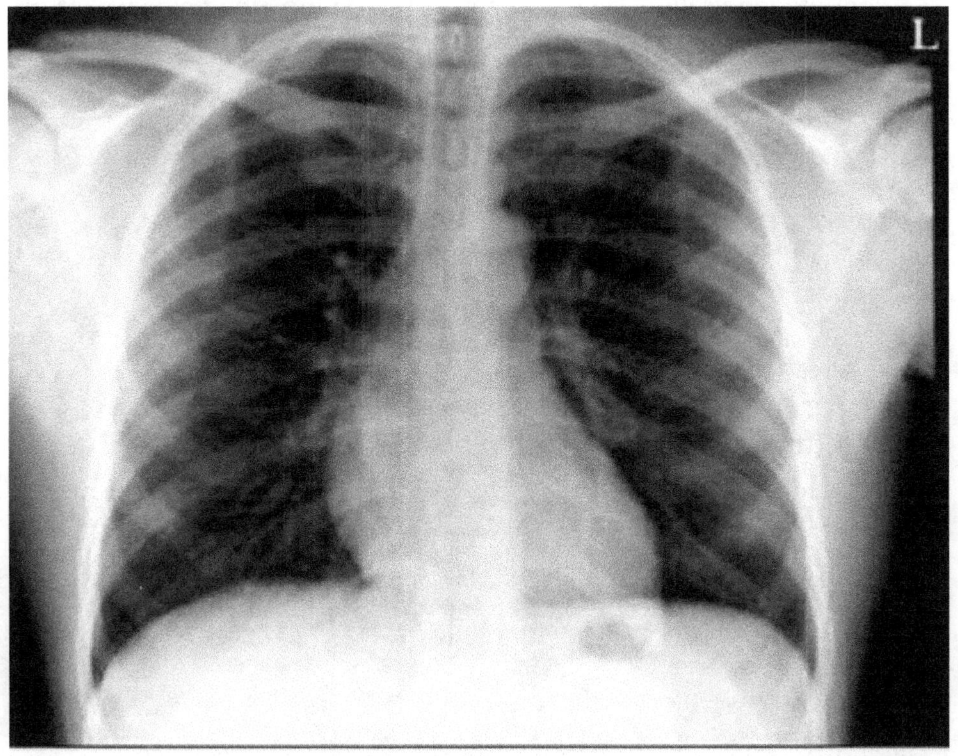

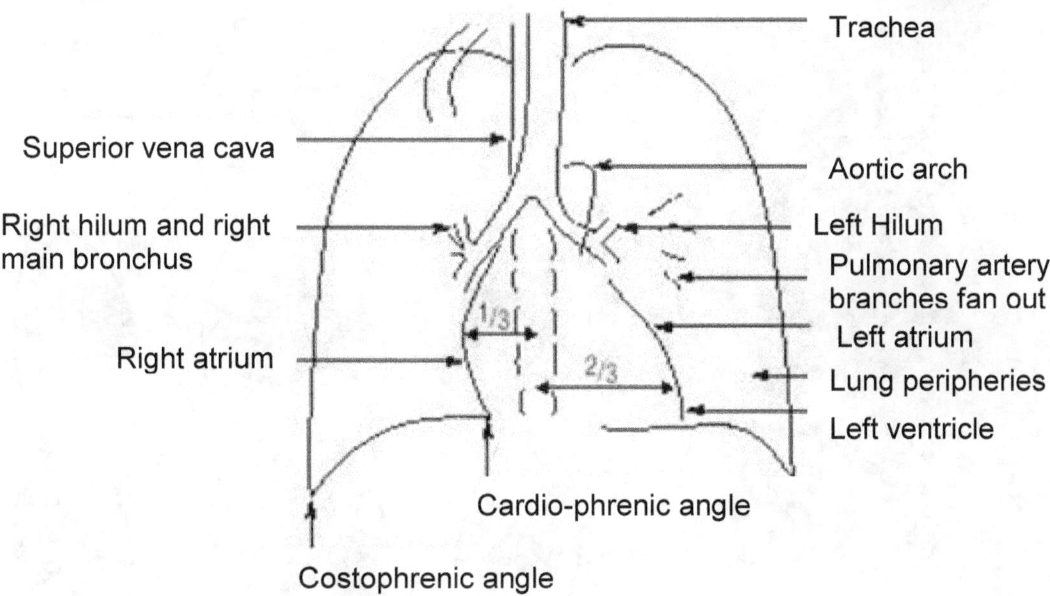

Provided through the courtesy of: Dr. A. Leung.

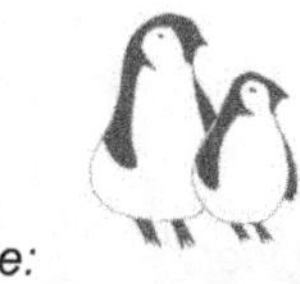

- Lung fields on inspiration, lobes and fissures.
    - Adequate inspiration - should be able to see the lung fields well: 6-8 anterior, 9-11 posterior; penetration: should be able to see the spine behind the heart.
    - Pay careful attention to the pulmonary lobes and fissures.

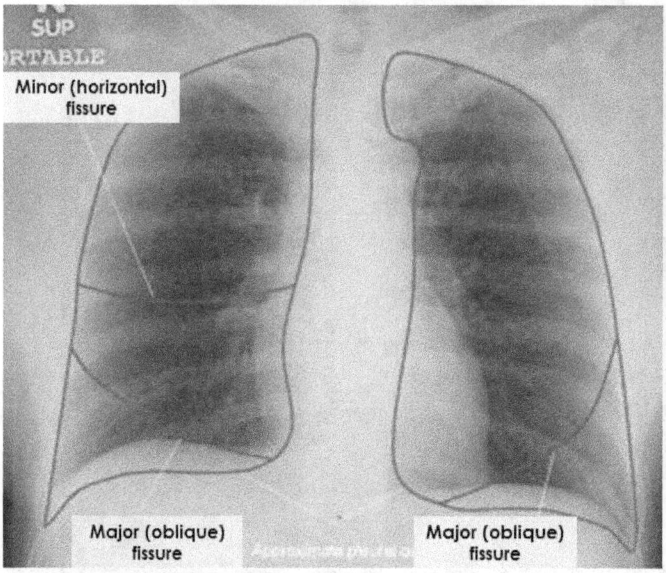

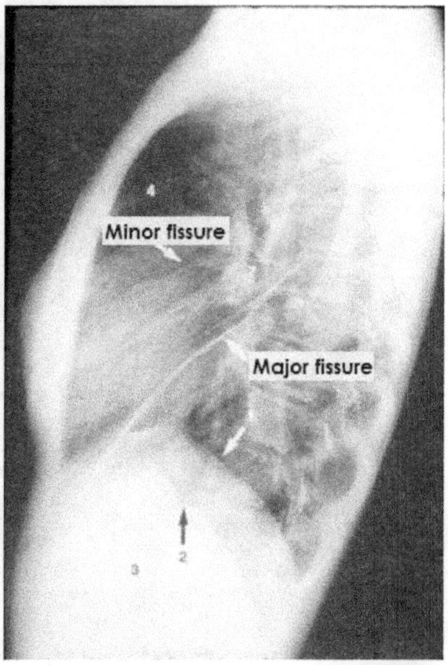

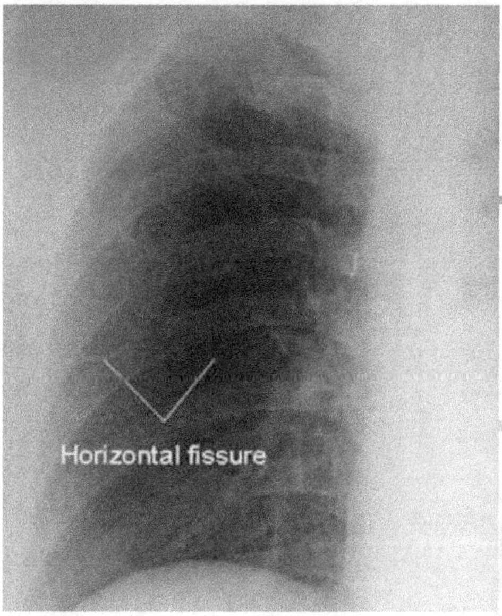

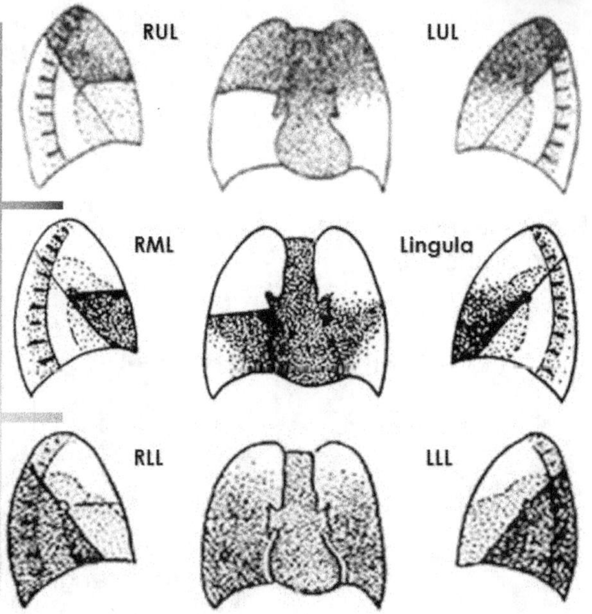

Provided through the courtesy of: Dr. A. Leung.

Example:

- Male patient. CXR.
- PA and lateral views.
- No date or name available.

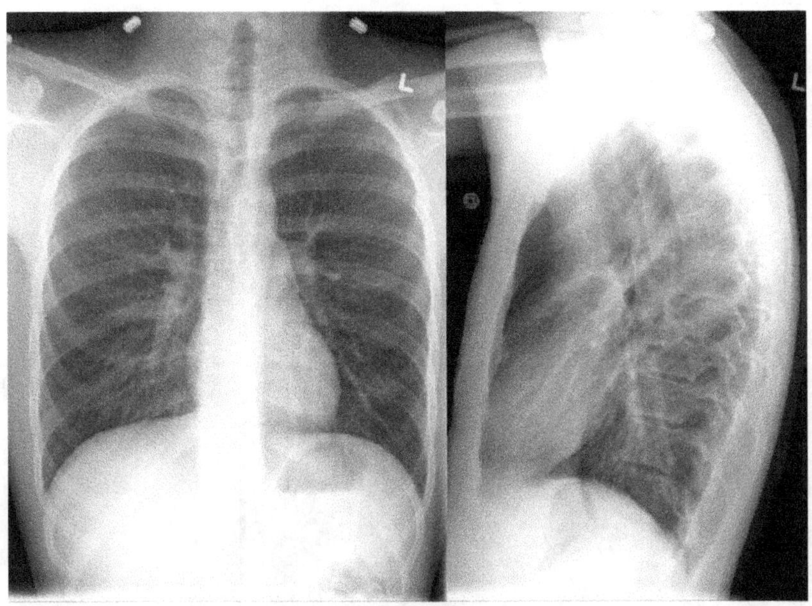

- The film is technically adequate
- Cardiac-thoracic ratio approximately 30%.
- No obvious cardiac chamber enlargement
- Right and left hilar contours preserved.
- No obvious lymphadenopathy, vessel enlargement, or masses.
- Normal AP window
- Contour of descending aorta normal
- Sharp costophrenic angles.
- Lung volumes preserved with normal lung markings.
- No obvious lung lesions or consolidative changes
- Soft tissue and bony structures normal
- Right hemidiaphragm slightly elevated.
- Gastric bubble noted inferior to left hemidiaphragm.

➢ Final diagnosis
  - Normal CXR.

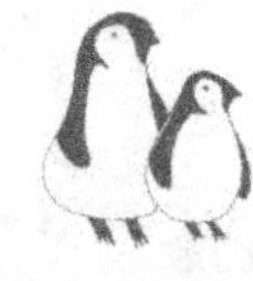

CASE STUDIES

Case one: Please describe the findings, give a differential, and state your most likely diagnosis.

- 75 year old man in ER with dyspnea

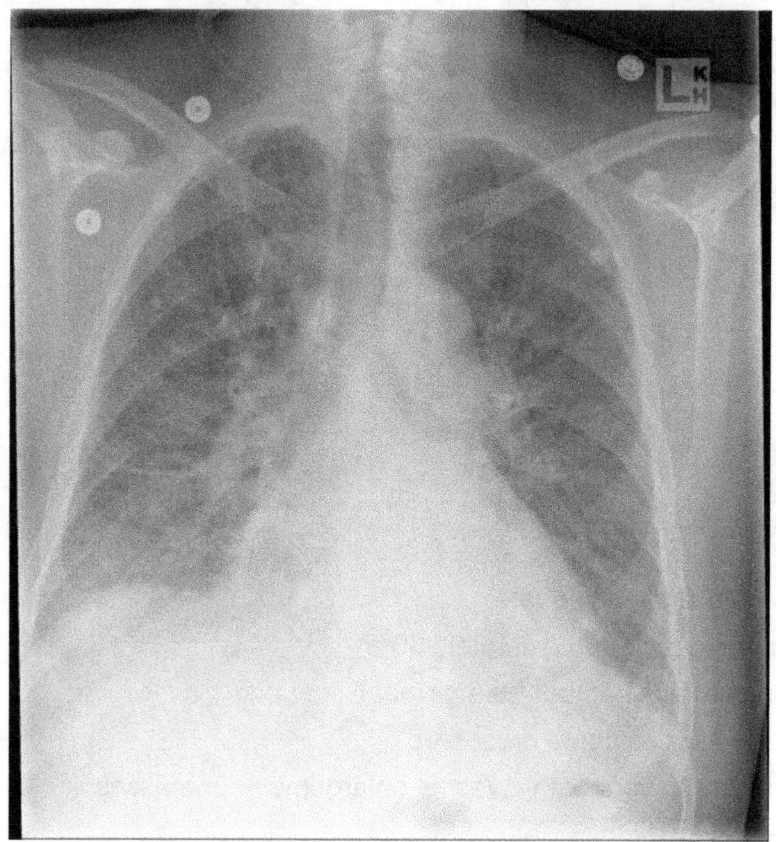

  - Interstial and airspace changes
  - Cardiomegaly
  - Ill-defined bronchovascular markings
  - Peribronchial cuffing;
  - Small pleural effusions
  - Fissural fluid and thickening

- Final diagnosis
  - Pulmonary interstitial edema

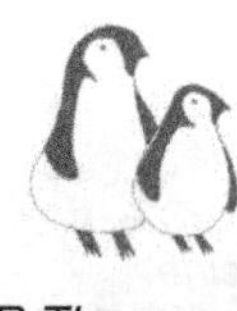

Case two: Please describe the findings, give a differential, and state your most likely diagnosis.

- No history given
    - Chest x-ray finding in the patient with congestive heart failure (CHF)
    - Kerley B & A septal lines
    - Fissure lines
    - Pleural effusions
    - Peribronchial cuffing
    - Consolidative changes (bat-wings appearance)
    - Vascular redistribution (cephalization)
    - Cardiomegaly

- Differential diagnosis
    - Pulmonary edema
    - Heart failure
    - Sepsis
    - Renal failure
    - ARDS
    - Lymphangitis carcinomatosis

Case three: Please describe the findings, give a differential, and state your most likely diagnosis.

- 29 year old with asthma presenting with dry cough

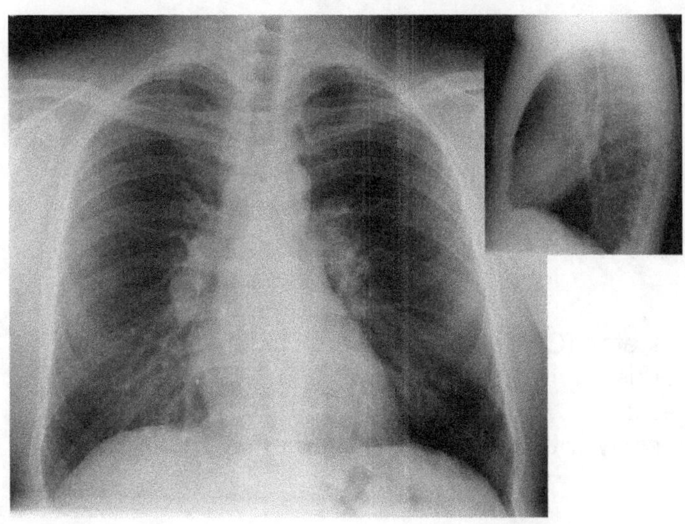

- Differential diagnosis of lymphadenopathy seen on chest x-ray
    - Sarcoidosis
    - TB
    - Cancer (mets and lymphoma)
    - Silicosis
    - Pulmonary hypertension

Case four: Please describe the findings, give a differential, and state your most likely diagnosis.

- 60 year old with worsening exertional dyspnea

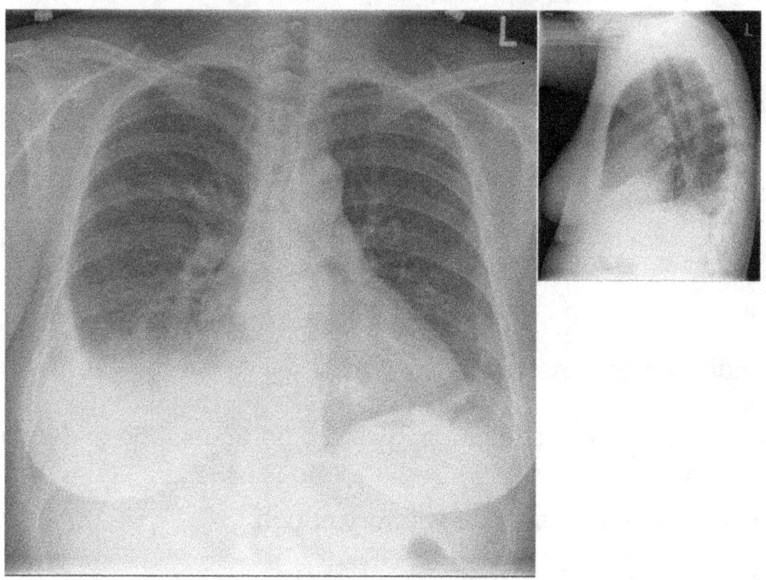

- Chest x-ray findings suggestive of pleural effusions
    - Blunted costophrenic angle
    - Opacification of diaphragm
    - Usually dependent, mobile, "meniscus" sign
    - Lateral view more sensitive
    - Supine: hazy 'veiling'

- Differential diagnosis
    - Volume overload states (CHF, cirrhosis, renal failure)
    - Parapneumonic effusion from pneumonia
    - Infections (empyema)
    - Malignancy (especially with isolated left-sided effusions)
    - Pancreatitis
    - Hypothyroidism

Case five: Please describe the findings, give a differential, and state your most likely diagnosis.

➢ 17 year old with asthma presenting with sudden dyspnea

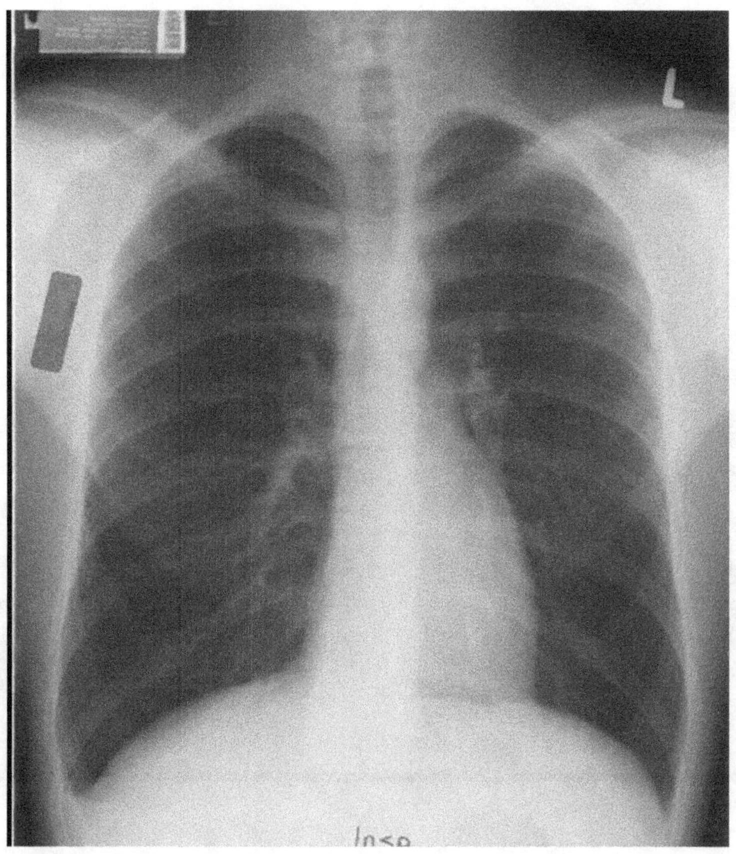

➢ Chest x-ray findings suggestive of pneumothorax
  - o Beware the normal CHX:
    - Always suspect a pneumothorax when you're given an x-ray on an exam that initially looks normal. With your finger, draw a very careful line around the pleural edges. Look for the following:
    - Pleural reflection **line**, no lung markings beyond
    - Sign of tension: mediastinal shift
  - o Pneumothoraces "pop-up" commonly on exams:
    - Young, thin & slim men with asthma...
    - Older men with a history of emphysema...
    - Mechanically ventilated patients with acute hypoxia...

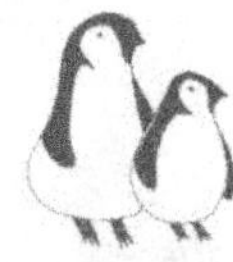

Case six: Please describe the findings, give a differential, and state your most likely diagnosis.

- Asymptomatic 40 year old 25-pack-year smoker

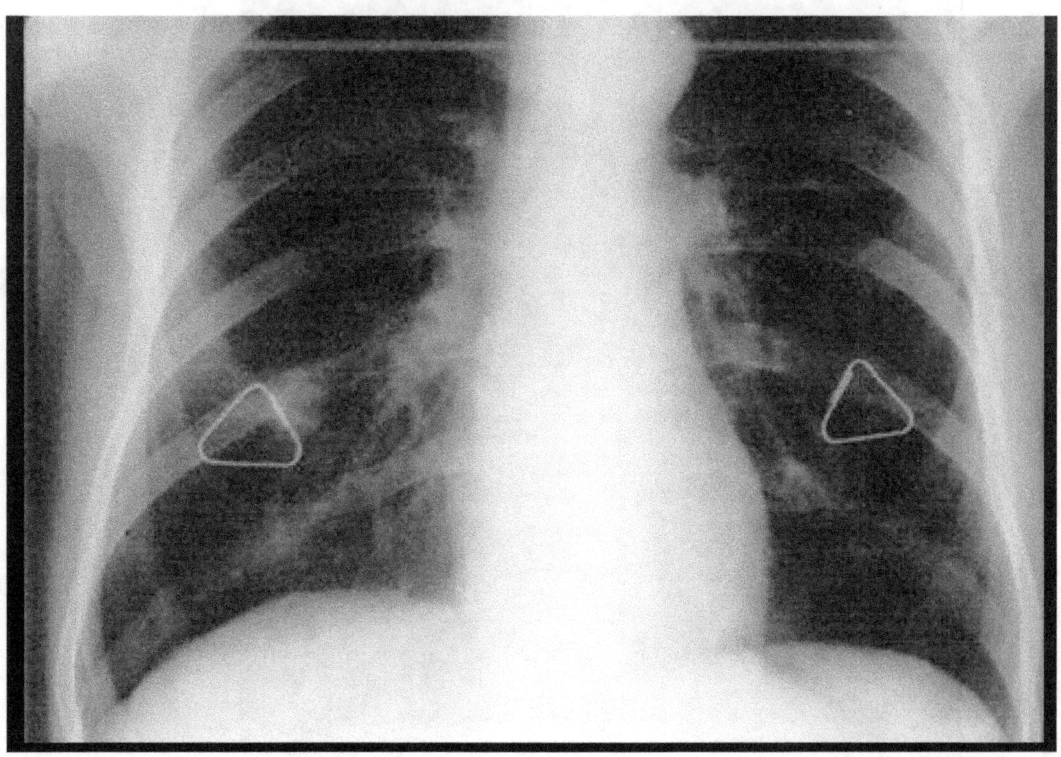

- Lung nodules seen on chest x-ray
    - Size & doubling time (< 30 days or > 2 years = good)
    - Borders (round & smooth = likely good; spiculated = likely bad)
    - Cavitation (necrosis)
    - Calcification (central/complete = TB/histoplasma; popcorn = benign)
    - Vascular markings (AVM)
    - Associated lesions/lymphadenopathy/collapse
    - Nodules < 3 cm; masses $\geq$ 3 cm in diameter

Case seven: Please describe the findings, give a differential, and state your most likely diagnosis.

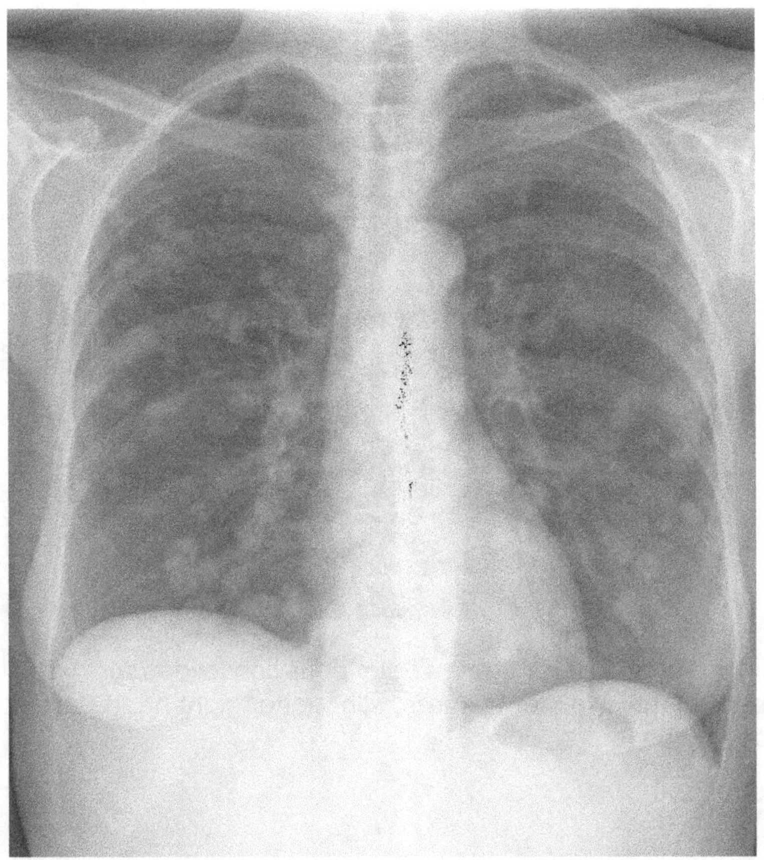

- Multiple lung nodules seen on chest x-ray
  - Neoplastic
    - Benign (hamartomas, cysts)
    - Malignant (mets, lymphoma, Kaposi sarcoma, bronchoalveolar cancer)
  - Infectious
    - Granulomas (TB, histoplasmosis)
    - Septic emboli
    - Viral pneumonias (measles, chickenpox)
  - Non-infectious, non-malignant
    - Rheumatoid nodules
    - Sarcoid
    - Wegener's granulomatosis
    - Infarcts
    - Round atelectasis

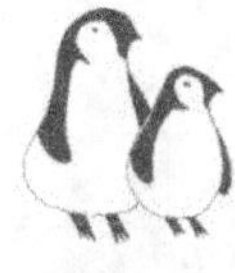

Case eight: Please describe the findings, give a differential, and state your most likely diagnosis.

- 50 year old with 3 day history of fever and chills, with productive cough

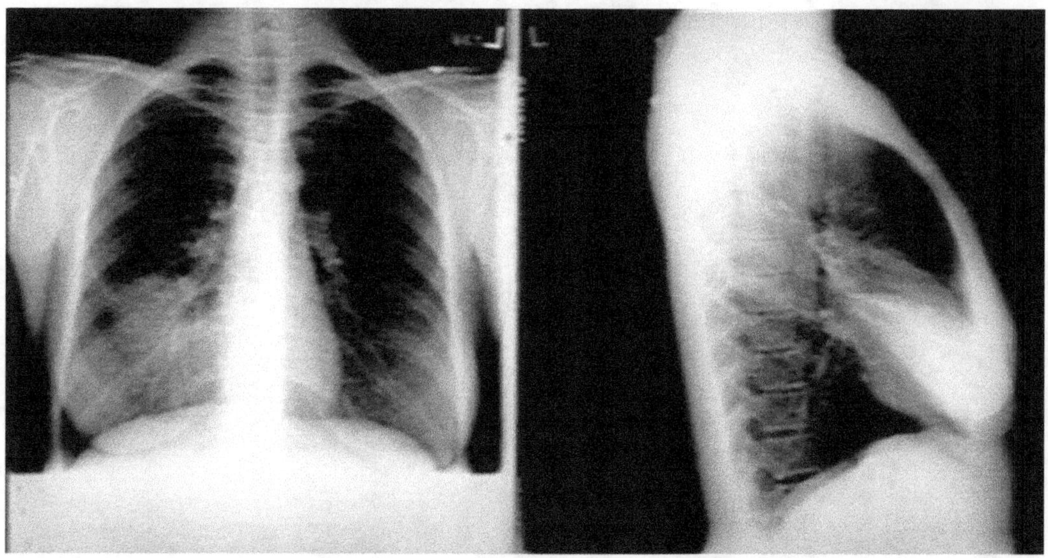

- Chest x-ray findings suggestive of right middle lobar consolidation
  - RML: abutment of major/minor fissures, silhouettes right heart border; easiest to identify on lateral view

- Differential diagnosis:
    - Infection
    - Aspiration
    - Tumour-mass
    - Tuberculosis
    - Interstitial pneumonia
  - Consolidation does not usually cause volume loss, unlike atelectasis; look at the fissure lines and surrounding structures for help(diaphragm and mediastinal structures)
  - Look for air bronchograms

- Chest x-ray findings suggestive of RML collapse
  - Right-sided volume loss
  - Hazy mid thoracic density obscuring right heart border
  - Wedge-shaped opacity on lateral film often not seen on frontal view except for volume loss with inferior displacement of minor fissure

➢ And worsens

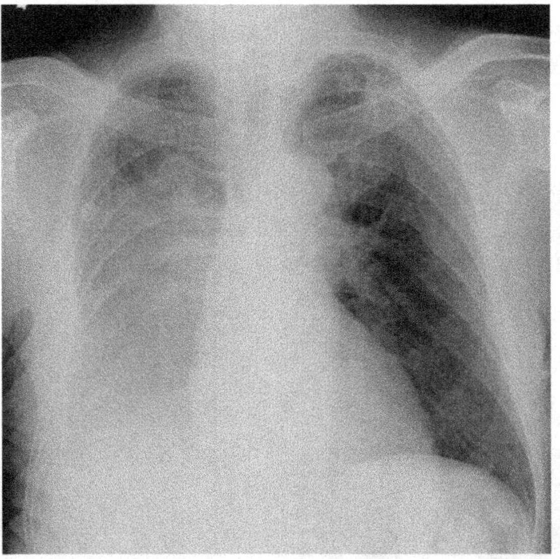

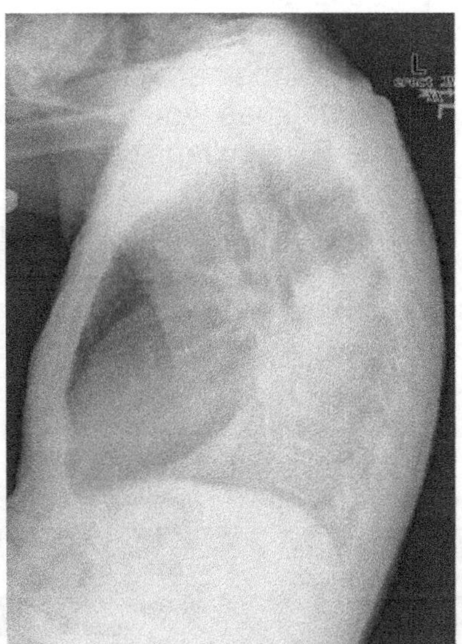

➢ Chest x-ray findings suggestive of RLL collapse and effusion
  - Lower and posterior zone opacity
  - Posterior displacement of major fissure
  - The right heart border is not obscured
  - The medial diaphragm is obscured

Case nine: Please describe the findings, give a differential, and state your most likely diagnosis.

➢ 70 year old with bronchiectasis presents with cough, dyspnea and pleuretic chest pain

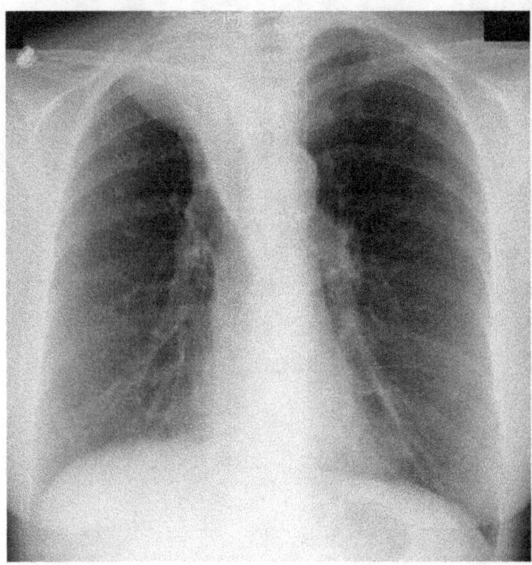

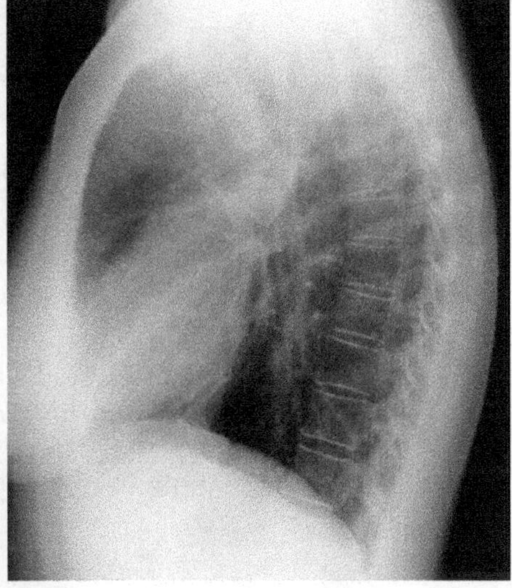

Chest x-ray findings suggestive of right upper lobar disease collapse

- Collapse
  - Elevation of minor fissure and right hilum
  - Wedge-shaped opacity at right lung apex
- Sometimes, you'll see the "Golden S sign" if there is a mass causing the RUL collapse
- Consolidation
  - Normal position of minor fissure

Case ten: Please describe the findings, give a differential, and state your most likely diagnosis.

- 30 year old with a 4 day history of cough and dyspnea

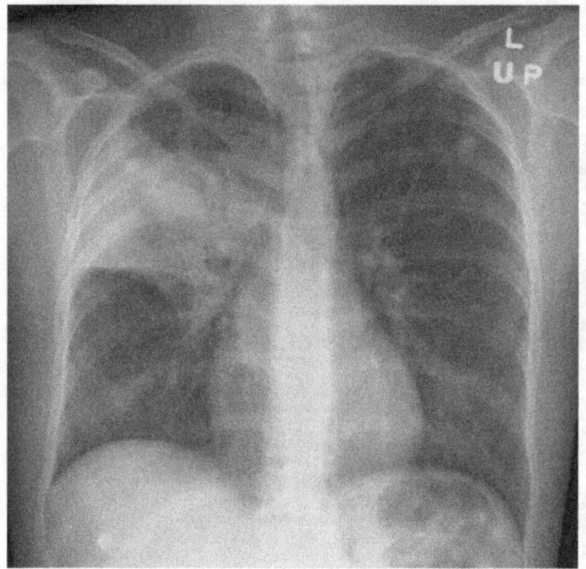

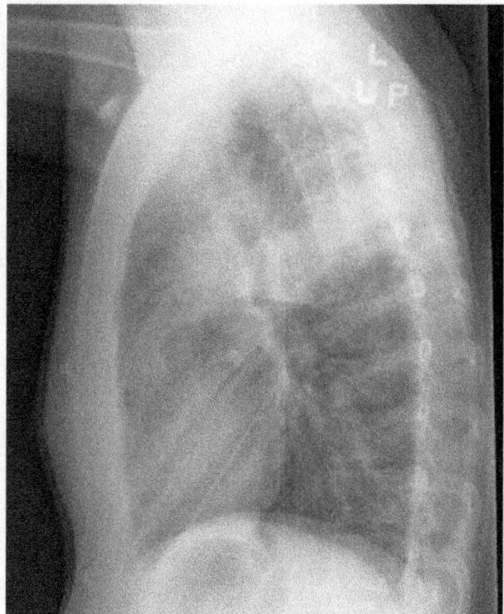

- Things to remember about right lobar consolidation
  - RML
    - Silhouettes right heart border
    - Easiest to see on lateral view
  - RLL
    - Difficult to differentiate from RML consolidation on PA film
    - Cardiac silhouette preserved
  - RUL
    - Look for triangle in right apex

Case eleven: Please describe the findings, give a differential, and state your most likely diagnosis.

- 65 year old with a 10 day history of productive cough, dyspnea and pleuritic chest pain

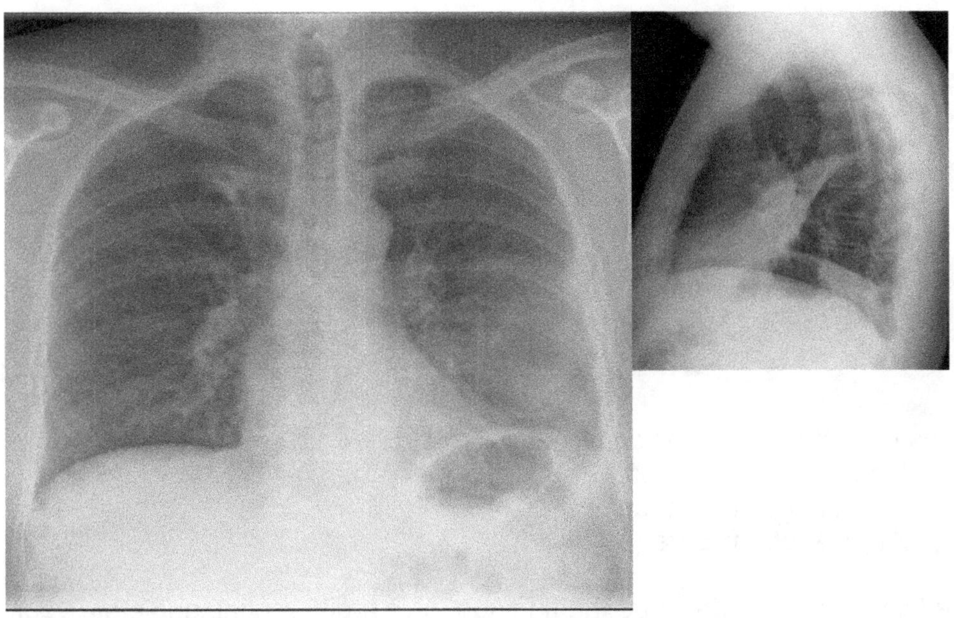

- Pay careful attention to the pulmonary lobes and fissures

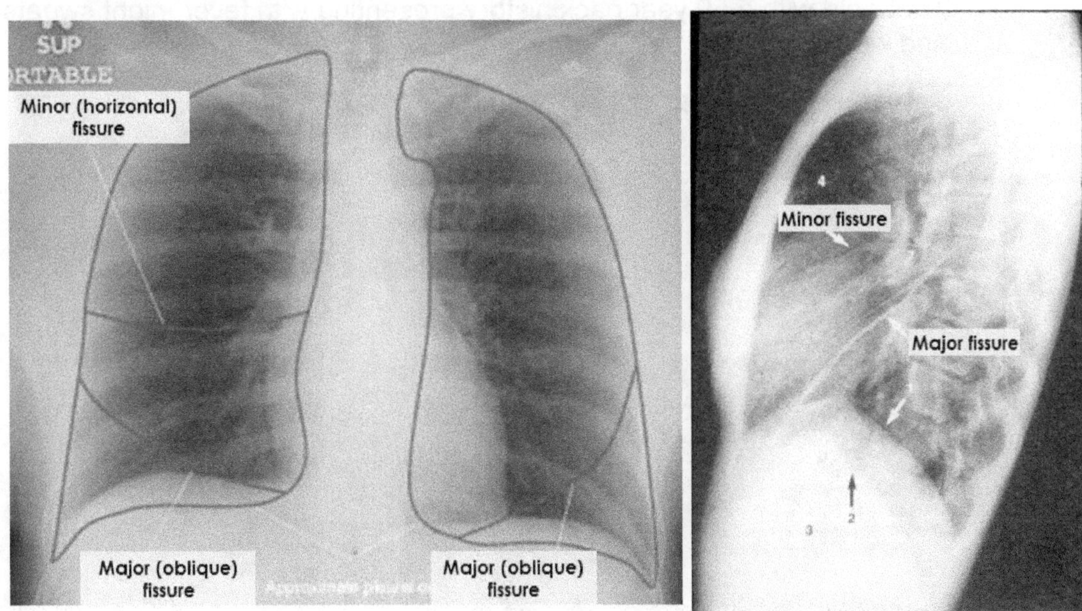

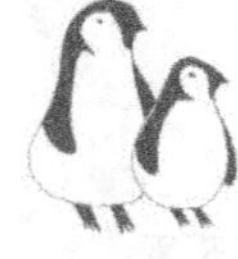

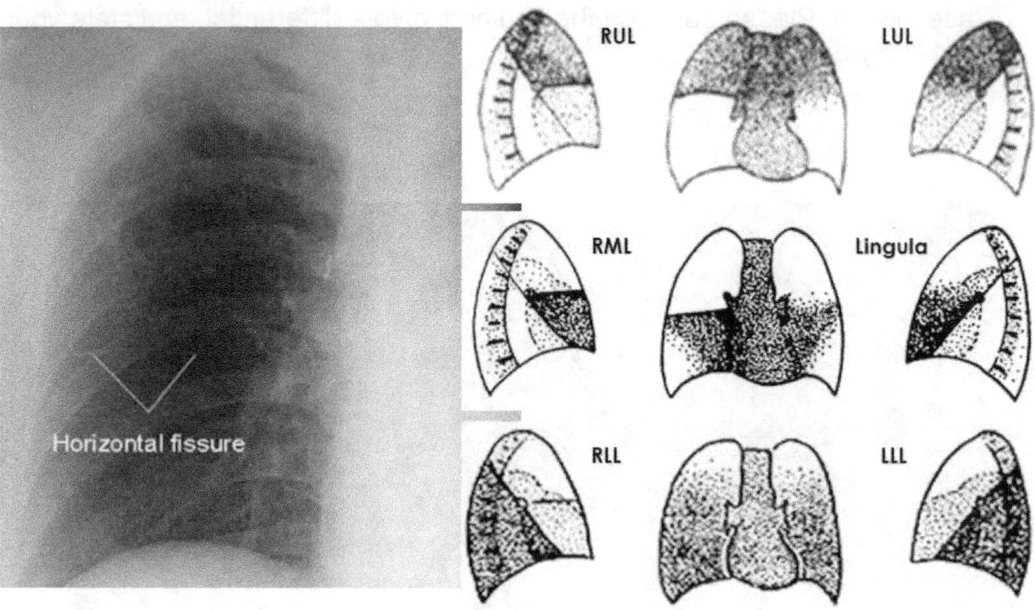

- This patient has lingular consolidation
    - Lingular consolidation
    - Small left pleural effusion
    - Azygos lobe fissure

Case twelve: Please describe the findings, give a differential, and state your most likely diagnosis.

- 80 year old with a 50 year pack history presenting with fever, night sweats and weight loss

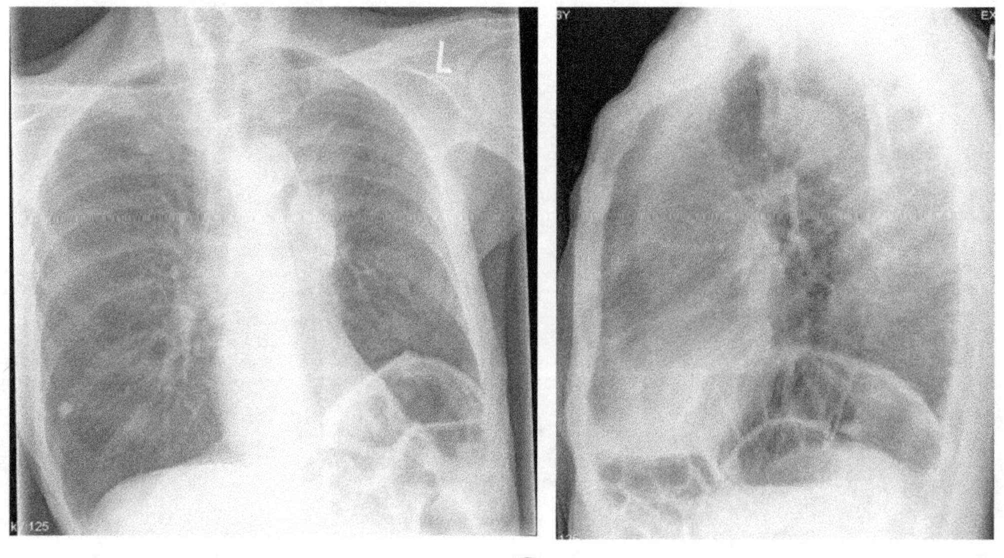

Chest x-ray findings suggestive of LUL collapse

- o The toughest one to diagnose
- o PA
  - Volume loss (elevation of L hemidiaphragm)
  - Luftsichel sign (LUL has retracted medically and superiorly. The hyperinflated LLL produces a crescent of lucency along the mediastinum and aortic knuckle)
- o Lateral
  - Anterior displacement of major fissure (// to sternum)
- o Golden S sign
  - Obstructing hilar mass (RUL or LUL)

(This man most likely has lung cancer with secondary LUL collapse)

Case thirteen: Please describe the findings, give a differential, and state your most likely diagnosis.

➢ 55 year involved in a MVA accident one year ago, when his CHX was normal

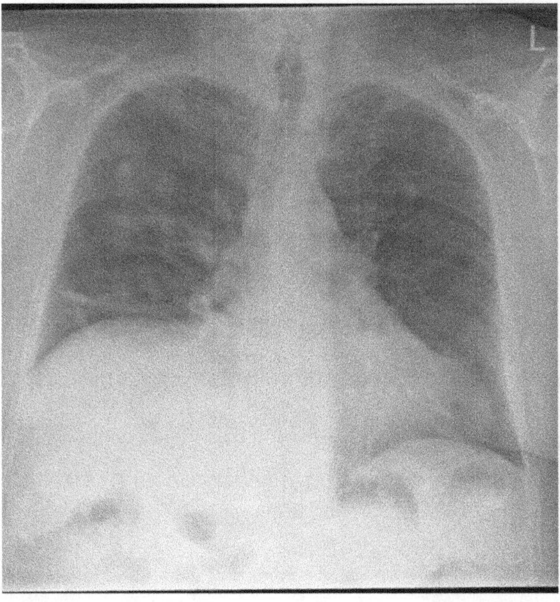

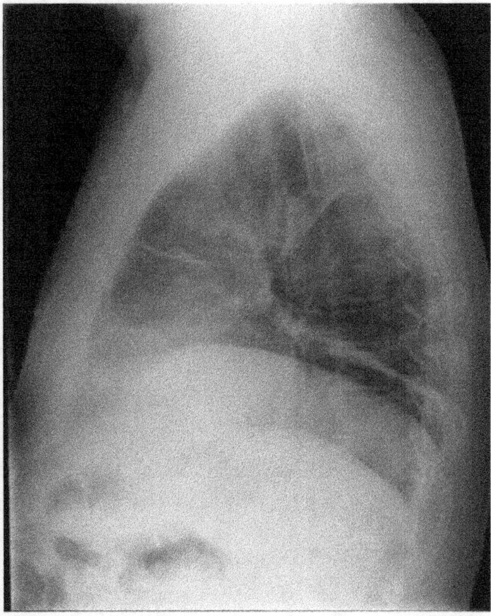

➢ Chest x-ray findings suggestive of elevation of a hemidiaphragm
  - o Normal R hemidiaphragm is ½ ICS higher than L in 90%
  - o DDX of elevated hemidiaphragm: The right hemidiaphragm is elevated

- Differential diagnosis
    - Diaphragmatic paralysis
    - Eventration of the diaphragm (R:L = 5.1)
    - Atelectasis
    - Subpulmonic effusion
    - Abdo disease (subphrenic abscess, liver mass, hernia)
    - Diaphragmatic rupture

Case fourteen: Please describe the findings, give a differential, and state your most likely diagnosis.

- "Routine" chest x-ray in a 55 year old asymptomatic woman with treated myasthemia gravis

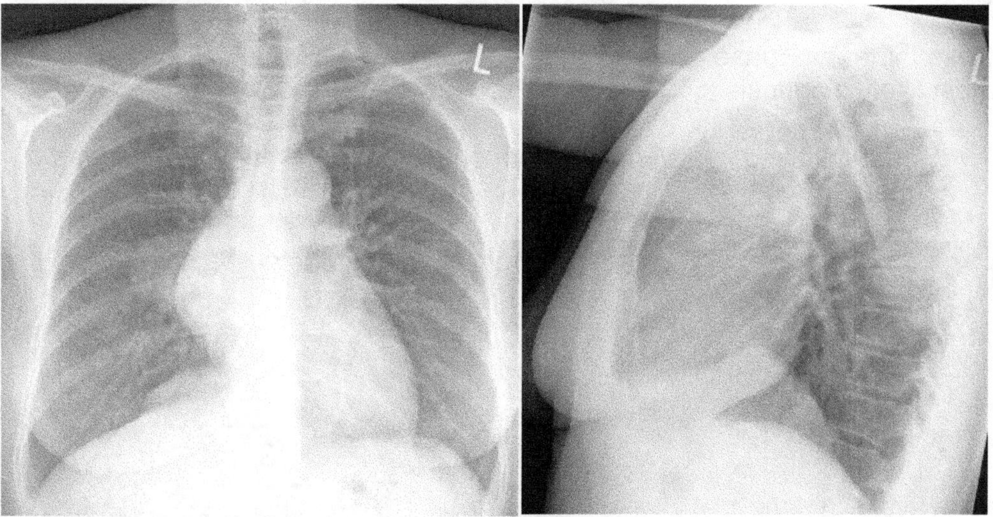

- Chest x-ray findings suggestive of anterior mediastinal masses
- If you are given an x-ray showing an anterior mediastinal mass, comment on:
    - Shape
    - Associated lung lesions (nodules, masses)
    - Surrounding structures (obscures ascending aorta, retrosternal airspace)
- Differential diagnosis (6 T's)
    - Thymoma
    - Thymic hyperplasia
    - Thyroid
    - Teratoma
    - Terrible lymphoma
    - Tumour

This lady also has a posterior mediastinal mass: final Dx turned out to be metastatic malignant thyomoma.

Case fifteen: Please describe the findings, give a differential, and state your most likely diagnosis.

- 50 year old homeless man with productive cough, decreased LOC and wasting

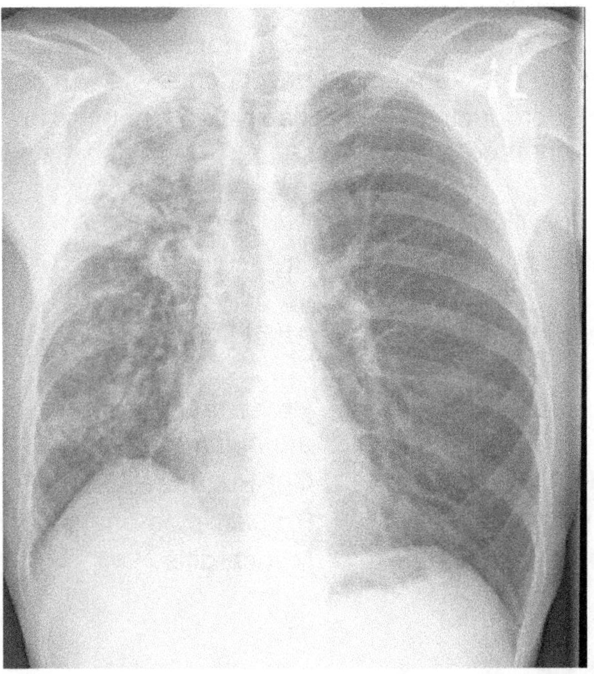

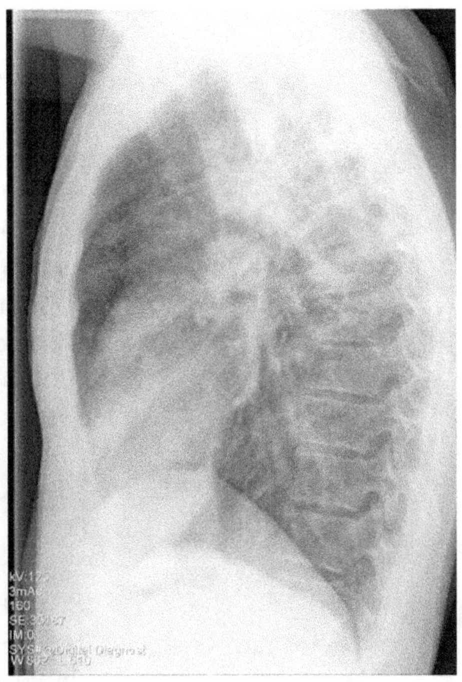

- Chest x-ray findings suggestive of apical fibrosis
    - Right sided volume loss with apical fibrosis
    - Right sided lung nodule with central cavitation
    - Right sided mediastinal lymphadenopathy

- Differential diagnosis
    - Active TB
    - Talcosis
    - Sarcoidosis
    - Fibrosis secondary to recurrent pneumonias

SUGGESTED PRACTICE CASE SCENARIOS FOR OSCE EXAMINATIONS

Primary Stem	Secondary Stem	Diagnosis
➢ Dyspnea	o Post operative	- Pulmonary embolism
	o Six week post acute MI	- CHF
	o With fever & productive cough in young person	- Community acquire pneumonia
	o With fever & productive cough in demented person	- Aspiration Pneumonia
	o With fever in MHSM	- Pneumocystis
	o With purulent sputum and clubbing	- Bronchiectasis/Cystic fibrosis
	o Acute onset in elderly person with palpitations	- Atrial fibrillation
	o Fever and pleural effusion	- Parapneumonic effusion/empyema
	o Advanced COPD	- Cor Pulmonale
	o Young person	- Primary pulmonary HTN
	o Exertional in young person	- Myocarditis
➢ Hemoptysis	o With fever in Asian immigrant	- TB
	o Chronic smoker	- Ca Lung
	o Chronic Smoker	- Bronchitis
	o With fever, epistaxis & renal failure	- Wegeners
➢ Abnormal CXR	o Young female with hot nodules in legs	- Sarcoidosis
➢ Chest X-ray	o Solitary pulmonary nodule in 68 yr old	- Ca Lung

Source: Kindly provided by Dr. P Hamilton (U of Alberta)

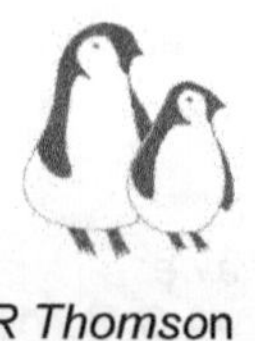

The "ABCs" of Reading a Chest X-Ray

- **A** – airway (midline, no obvious deformities, no paratracheal masses).
- **B** – bones and soft tissue (no fractures, subcutaneous emphysema).
- **C** – cardiac size, silhouette, and retrocardiac density normal.
- **D** – diaphragms (right above left by 1cm to 3cm, costophrenic angles sharp, diaphragmatic contrast with lung sharp).
- **E** – equal volume 9count ribs, look for mediastinal shift).
- **F** – fine detail (pleura and lung parenchyma).
- **G** – gastric bubble (above the air bubble one shouldn't see an opacity of any more than 0.5cm width).
- **H** – hilum (left normally above right by up to 3cm, no larger than a thumb), hardware (in the intensive care unit: endotracheal tube, central venous catheters).

"Science is never cast in stone and ideas are written with a finger on shifting sand."

Anonymous

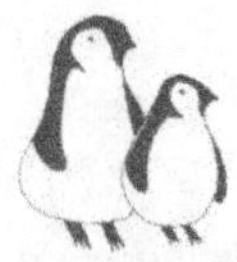

ONLINE RESOURCES:

- MedEdPORTAL: https://www.mededportal.org/
- Portal of online geriatric education: http://www.pogoe.org/
- AGA educator resources: http://www.gastro.org/gi-fellowship/educator-resources
- http://www.gastro.org/practive/medical-osition-statements
- Home parenteral Nutrition: www.oley.org
- Intestinal transplantation: http://www.intestinaltransplant.org
- CCFA: http://www.ccfa.org
- CCFC (Crohn's and Colitis Foundation of Canada): www.ccfc.ca
- http://www.pathology.pitt.edu/lectures/gi
- www.orl.cz/ehorroby/ustni/vestibulum/veozena
- http://www.pathologyatlas.com
- http://www.mayoclinic.org/gi-risk/mayomodel2.html
- http://mayoclini.org/meld/mayomodel6.html
- www.gastro.org/practice/meicacl-osition-statements
- Natural Comprehensive Cancer Network (NCCN) guidelines: www.nccn.org
- http://www.accessdata.fda.gov/drugsatfda docs/label/2011/201917lbl.pdf
- http://www.accessdata.fda.gov/drugsatfda docs/label/2011/201917lbl.pdf
- http://www.aidsinfo.nih.gov/guidelines/
- http://www.fda.gov/Drugs/DrugSafety/ucm291119.htm
- http://www.fda.gov/Drugs/DrugSafety/ucm291119.htm
- http://www.fda.gov/NewsEvents/Newsroom/PressAnnouncements/ucm256299.htm
- http://www.fda.gov/Safety/MedWatch/SafetyInformation/SafetyAlertsforHumanMedicalProducts/ucm291144.htm
- http://www.fda.gov/Safety/MedWatch/SafetyInformation/SafetyAlertsforHumanMedicalProducts/ucm211796.htm
- www.aasid.org/practiceguidelines/Page/default.aspx
- http://www.accessdata.fda.gov/drugsatfda does/label/2011/201917lbl.pdf

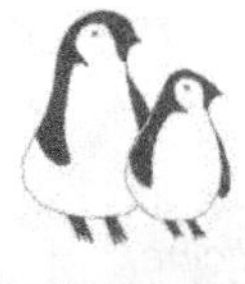

- www.aasld.org/practiceguidelines/Page/default.aspx
- National Endoscopy Program : www.grs.nhs.uk
- *MELD, Model for End-Stage Liver Disease, available online calculator: www.mayoclinic.org/meld/mayomodel7.html
- www.motherisk.org/women/index.jsp
- National Endoscopy Program : www.grs.nhs.uk
- CAPstone: http://www.giandhepatology.com
- MedicineNet: www.medicinenet.com/irritable_bowel_syndrome/article.htm
- IBS Support group: www.ibsgroup.org
- UpdateToDate: www.uptodate.com/patients/index
- International Association for the Study of Obesity: http://www.iaso.org
- Liver and intrahepatic bile ducts. www.PathologyOutlines.com
- Medical council of Canada. Weight Gain/Obesity. http://mcc.ca/Objectives_Online/
- Medical Council of Canada. Weight Loss/ Eating Disorders/ Anorexia http://mcc.ca/Objectives_Online/
- Medical council of Canada. Weight loss/Eating Disorders/Anorexia. http://mcc.ca/Objectives_Online/
- http://www.fda.gov/Drugs/DrugSafety/PostmarketDrugSafetyInformationforPatientsandProviders/ucm213038.htm.
- Me'decins San Frontieres: http://www.msf.org
- Recommendations about chemoprophylaxis for malaria. Also see http://www.nc.cdc.gov/travel/yellowbook/2012/chapter-3-infectious-disease-related-to-travel/malaria.htm

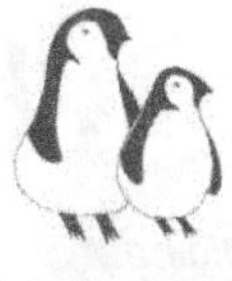

INDEX

Note: Page number followed by f and t indicates figure and table respectively.

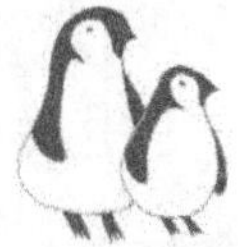

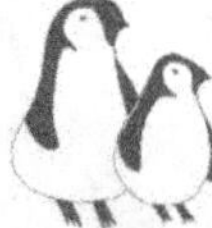

B

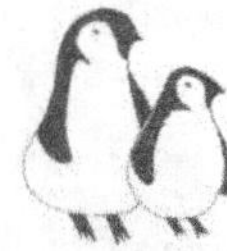

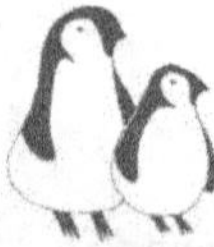

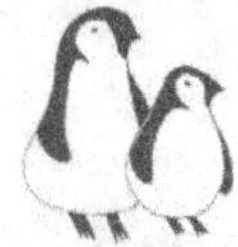

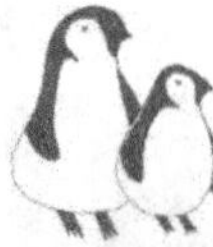

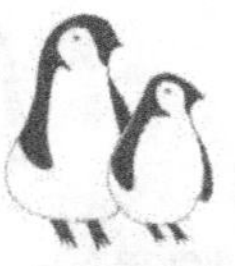

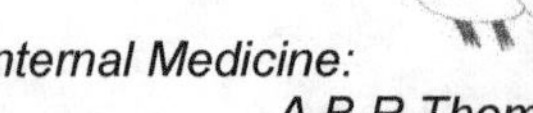

G

H

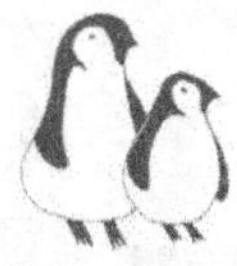

I

K

L

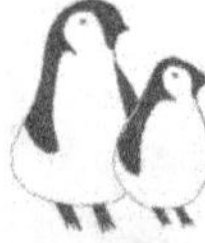

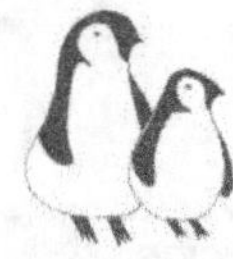

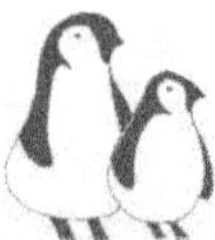

N

O

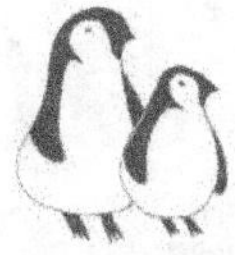

P

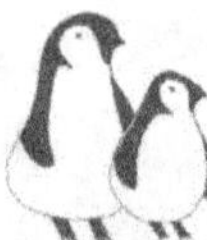

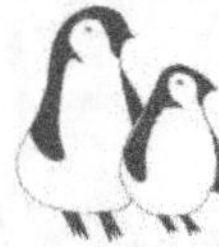

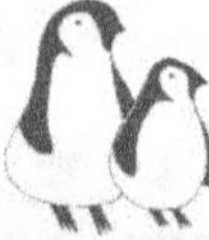

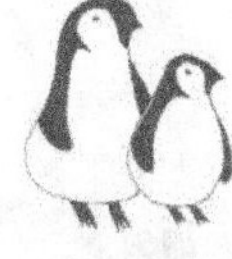

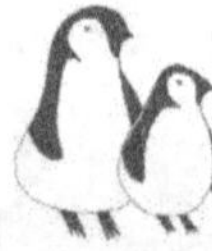

T

U

V

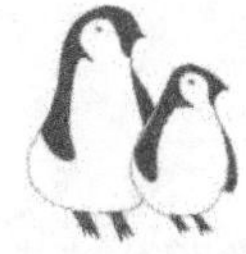

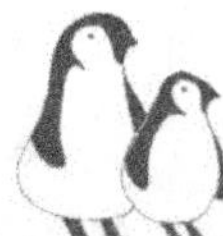